SWINE FLU: PANDEMIC STRIKES

The New H1N1 Threat

Compiled and Edited by
Sunaina Chaturvedi

Foreword by
Maj Gen Raj Mehta

PENTAGON PRESS

Swine Flu: Pandemic Strikes / Sunaina Chaturvedi (Ed)

ISBN 978-81-8274-431-8

First Indian Edition 2009

Published by

PENTAGON PRESS
206, Peacock Lane, Shahpur Jat, New Delhi-110049
Phones: 011-64706243, 26491568
Telefax: 011-26490600
email: rajan@pentagon-press.com
website: www.pentagon-press.com

Printed at

New Elegant Printers
New Delhi, India.

Foreword

When the breaking news story of the outbreak of Swine Flu in Mexico took place on March 18 this year, I was only mildly curious. Mexico was too far away to affect my daily life, I thought. This disease is some one else's headache, not mine, I smugly rationalised. In any case, this is a disease of the Americas; it cannot possibly reach India for a decade yet, I assured myself.

It did. The first confirmed case of Swine Flu was reported in India, on May 16, 2009. It was a 23 year old US based NRI returning from USA, who was detected with it during thermal screening conducted at Hyderabad International Airport. The first unfortunate victim of the virus, a 14 year old school girl from Pune, Rida Ayesha Shaikh, died on August 4, 2009, after alleged mishandling of her diagnosis and treatment by two private hospitals. She had developed symptoms on July 21, which were apparently misinterpreted by those treating her.

The speed with which the virus (and knowledge about it) has spread in an increasingly interconnected world need not really have surprised me. I remembered reading Thomas Friedman's *'The World is Flat'* in 2005, and had agreed whole heartedly with its basic premise of a *flat* world, a word, which Friedman found prescient and which forms the title of his book. Friedman recounts a conversation with Nandan Nilekani (former CEO, Infosys) during which Nilekani made him realise that the world is "flat," in the sense that globalization has leveled the playing fields between industrial and emerging countries (such as India). In his opinion, this flattening is a product of a convergence of personal computer with fiber-optic micro cable with the rise of workflow (the ability of a machine to talk to a machine without human interference) software.

Friedman defined ten "flatteners" that he saw as leveling the global playing field. Of these ten, two need to be quoted because of the manner in which they have affected the spread of information on H1N1 2009 Flu, and, indirectly, its possible, eventual management and control.

- **Flattener #9: In-forming**: Google and other search engines are the prime example. "Never before in the history of the planet have so many people-on their own-had the ability to find so much information about so many things and about so many other people", writes Friedman. The growth of search engines is tremendous; for example take Google, in which Friedman states that it is "now processing roughly one billion searches per day, up from 150 million just three years ago".
- **Flattener #10: "The Steroids"**: Personal digital devices like mobile phones, iPods, personal digital assistants, instant messaging, and voice over Internet Protocol (VoIP).

The terrifying speed with which the virus has spread worldwide and reached India in less than three months of its identification in Mexico is obviously not attributable to Friedman's thesis, but to the macabre characteristics of the virus. The speed at which an avalanche of information about the virus has criss-crossed the world is, however, certainly attributable to his understanding of how the above flatteners have impacted on the spread of information, and, therefore, knowledge to combat H1N1 Flu 2009. This is one lesson that I feel the common man, *everyman*, Governments, organizations have probably learnt from the electrifying manner in which this "Americas' disease has, almost overnight, become a true pandemic, affecting all nations of the world.

Wikipedia reports that this 2009 Flu pandemic is a truly global outbreak of a new strain of influenza virus. It was officially named the **"new H1N1"**, first identified in March 2009, and is commonly (and mistakenly) called the "Swine Flu." It is thought to be a mutation of four known strains of the **Influenza A** virus, subtype H1N1: one endemic in (normally infecting) humans, one endemic in birds, and two endemic in pigs (swine). Influenza A virus strains have caused three major global epidemics during the 20th century: the 'Spanish' flu in 1918, Asian flu in 1957 and Hong Kong flu in 1968–69.

It is worth objectively recording, at this stage, the trauma that this virus caused in its first avatar, when it surfaced as "Spanish Flu'. It was caused by an unusually virulent and deadly Influenza A virus strain of sub type H1N1 – an exact replica of the virus strain of the current pandemic. Understandably, neither the medical world, the public or, for that matter, the Governments who were then enmeshed in World War I, had much of an idea on what the virus could do, and how rapidly it could spread into a global disease; a pandemic. No wonder then, that in its life span of March 1918 to June 1920, it is responsible for having killed between 50 to a 100 million people worldwide.

The current 2009 virus was first reported in two American children on March 18, 2009. Some experts now assume that Mexico already had hundreds of thousands, and possibly millions, of cases before the outbreak was officially recognized, and were therefore in the midst of a "silent epidemic." Experts agree that the new virus is a type of swine influenza, derived originally from a strain that lived in pigs. This origin gave rise to the common name of "swine flu", largely used by mass media. *Despite this origin, however, the current strain is transmitted between people and not from swine.* The initial panic reaction of banning pork imports, mass extermination of pigs (swine) and blanket bans on eating pork are, therefore, not justified and many countries have recalled their restrictions in this sphere.

On June 11, 2009, the WHO declared the outbreak had become a pandemic. On a separate scale for severity, WHO has assessed the global severity as "moderate." 221,591 people have been affected worldwide and 2123 people had died of Swine Flu infection as of 15 August 2009. In India, those affected had crossed 1400 on the same date, with deaths pegged at 26.

The statistics, by comparison, of some other countries in this regard are revealing. A short list is given below:

Mexico	Affected 18,861	Dead 163
USA	Affected 46,752	Dead 450
Hong Kong	Affected 6,640	Dead 4
Israel	Affected 2,148	Dead 8
Vietnam	Affected 1300	Dead 2

It is quite clear that observance of due precautions, adequate and well equipped diagnostic centres, speedy, hassle free and correct diagnosis and follow up treatment, post treatment and cure precautions to avoid recurrence, as well as spread of knowledge and information across the board about all aspects of the virus finds reflection in the fatalities suffered.

A growing number of people are critical of Governance in India, as also of our apex medical authorities and bureaucrats for being caught off guard yet again. This is what they have concluded, particularly after the Government had, since May 2009, been assuring the nation that it was carrying out "effective screening" at all points of entry (presumably major airports and sea ports), and was fully prepared for all exigencies. The critics contend that this claim fell flat with the first viral death at Pune and investigation of serious lapses and lack of coordination thereof by a proactive media.

The investigations and subsequent Government admission revealed how ill prepared the nation actually was. Editorial comment in some newspapers has taken the Union Health Minister to task for not being able to put his act together and failing to provide proper guidance and check back on the actual state of the nation's preparedness. The bureaucrats have, very correctly, not escaped censure for failing to implement the procedures, checks and balances; in fact, for failure to create, sustain and monitor a robust, credible action plan to combat the virus, incorporating the lessons learnt from the mistakes made by countries in the West and South America. They contend that this all round mental paralysis and absence of an overall vision, the strategy to implement it as also the need to manage public perceptions by keeping the public informed to prevent panic not only in the lay public but also those diagnosed as suffering from Swine Flu 2009 (H1N1 strain) reveals how badly off we actually are.

This is where I have an opportunity as well as a professional obligation to explain why I, a person who does not have more than passing knowledge of the virus (gleaned primarily from the internet and conversations with doctor and paramedical friends, one of them a gritty, knowledgeable Scottish lady medical practitioner, who, along with her Professor husband, were on FLAME rolls till recently) has been requisitioned to write the Foreword of this topical and most needed book.

Firstly, I was shocked by the death of the young school girl at Pune; more so because I am a Visiting Faculty at an upcoming educational Institute at Pune, the Foundation for Liberal And Management Education (FLAME). The emotional bonding with the children and my understanding of my social responsibilities stung me into immediate action, compelling me to read up on the disease (remember, it is a *flat* world, where you have instant access to quality information; thereby knowledge) and send a two page note to the Chairman and President of FLAME on the day little Rida Ayesha Shaikh died. They ensured its reproduction on the FLAME portal without delay, and passed monitorable instructions for its implementation.

Secondly, I see the virus issue as a problem that needs a time sensitive, full spectrum execution. I am not at all overwhelmed to see this outbreak as a critical generalist tasking for which I should clearly see what needs resolution and then put down succinctly how this is to be done, leaving all technical and medical execution details for those who are trained for it. Surely this was what the country may have expected of the Health Minister and the bureaucrats of his ministry.

Since criticism especially in a growing, nascent democracy is endemic and everyone's birthright, one must put a stop to it and, instead, turn to positive and useful suggestions and recommendations. There is also both merit and maturity in accepting that mistakes have been made that do not need repetition and moving on.

The simple but effective approach to problem resolution is to ask three simple questions and then seek their answers logically and thoroughly. This is called the "Appreciation process" and involves asking the questions: What is my task? What does it involve? And, lastly, how far can I plan now?

The task is simple – or, at least seems so. One is tempted to say, "Eliminate the H1N1 2009 Swine Flu virus from India". This, is, however, patently wrong tasking. The virus is already a pandemic. At best, it can now only be contained. A better tasking would be "Avoid Mortality". A secondary, spin off task is obviously, "Contain contagion". This will mean a review of our entire systems and wherewithal to save lives; public/private hospital coordination for diagnostics, provision of knowledge, doctors and technicians, adequate, well equipped diagnostic centres testing kits, infrastructure that can be isolated, medicine, et al.

The second question (what does it involve?) is also easily answered. It involves a total overhaul of the current, piecemeal approach, and its replacement by a synergized, all encompassing, holistic approach that runs across the entire gamut of fighting the Swine Flu virus from its clear identification till its elimination from affected patients (remember the clear tasking: "Avoid Mortality"?). The spin off tasking of "Containing contagion" is equally comprehensively tackled by setting into motion all medical and technical checks and balances applicable to India, culled from our own exposure as well as from lessons learnt from countries who have suffered this virus earlier than us. Here, medical advice tendered by WHO, CDC and other knowledgeable bodies should also be dovetailed. Containing contagion will also be a function of strict 24×7 manning of all entry points; not just at airports and sea ports but also along national borders that are land based and where people transit such as at Wagah, trade check posts in Kashmir, in North Sikkim, along the Indo Bangladesh and Indo Burmese, Indo Nepalese, Indo Bhutan borders.

The world over, what is used for screening is thermal cameras/ machines that detect human body temperatures above 39 degrees centigrade and then check the isolated patients for respiratory distress and fever record. There is also need for carrying out Active as opposed to Passive data collection. The Active method of data collection targets the target population by stratified random sampling, which is considered much more effective.

There is also need to carry out properly controlled epidemiological studies of the 2009 virus outbreak in India. If these have been attempted in India, the public is not in the know. The need for wide spread education of the urban and rural masses, of people across the social divide in coping with the virus is most important and cannot be overstated. The issue of self medication (when not affected) by taking Tamiflu has already resulted in a resistant virus in a woman patient in Japan, on July 2, 2009. The prevention of prophylactic consumption of Tamiflu and Relenza by people with over the counter access to these drugs will render all such treatment useless and complicate treatment of the virus enormously. It is a medical as well as social obligation of Government to prevent this from happening.

The last question is regarding the planning process (How far can I plan now?). It would be a good idea to focus on not only creating a vaccine to suit Indian conditions, which will allow for protecting a large portion of the target population that can catch the virus, but also creating it in sync with similar efforts going on the world over. It is believed that a vaccine made by the Swiss pharma firm, Novartis is already under trial at Costa Rica since July 31, 2009 and US and UK are about to start their vaccine trials. Consolidation of such knowledge will stop us from wasting time in reinventing the wheel.

The appreciation process, the lay reader will agree, is thus a simple yet holistic process that a leader, political or otherwise can implement and monitor. The fact that one is not a doctor does not disqualify from setting up such a process in motion and then assiduously monitoring it until completion. It is a sterling exposition; another name for the classic Clauzewitzian formula of *Ends, Ways* and *Means*. The national leadership; in fact, leadership at all levels in particular and the working level leadership in general needs its clear understanding and ruthless implementation. The desired End (the objective) is that we must

"Avoid Mortality"—not lose any more citizens to this malaise. Apologies will not get Rida back for us. Only focused, synergized work will prevent future catastrophe. The Ways (method of work) and the Means (Resources needed/ best use of those available) have been explained clearly in the Appreciation process.

This timely book has been taken out with concern and understanding for the common man by Pentagon Press, and is in line with the urgent need to educate all strata of our 1.3 billion population, from medical professionals, people working in the public space, whether in politics, in Government departments, in NGO's to the *aam aadmi,* on the enormous viral challenges we face. A study of its contents reveals that every aspect of useful information on Swine Flu has been covered, including a chapter on what may be termed as *traditional Indian medical responses* in coping with variants of the Flu virus including the H1N1 virus. It is my considered opinion that the book bridges a serious, existing void in basic knowledge about the pandemic and how to cope with its control when it is suspected contacted or spread.

It is a handbook that should be available on call in educational institutions both public and private, in offices, at homes, with NGO's, with our uniformed forces, scientists, NRIs, immigration and customs offices, with the medical fraternity as well as in the corporate work place.

15 August 2009 **Raj Mehta**

Preface

Disease in the world is not uncommon. Even in the best of times in this world (sadly, which seemed to have passed), the one debilitating factor which all of us have been weary of has been disease; its nature and what it does to the one it infects.

Forever now, history has borne witness to outbreak upon outbreak of newer diseases, which have not just harmed our being, but also all that upon which we depend. For example, the Irish Famine wiped out potatoes, leading to mass starvation; or the outbreak of small pox which killed many, while disfiguring those fortunate enough to survive. And of course, the outbreak of plague which earned itself the unfortunate name of 'black death.'

It is not surprising that these outbreaks were never understood because the agents of these diseases were not visible. It was only when *Anton Van Leuwenhoek* invented the microscope in the late 17th century did we get a glimpse into the lives of these micro creatures.

These microcreatures are highly varied; in their structures, nature, their modes of causing disease, and even the way they reproduce. One of the most interesting of these have been viruses, which had been undetected untill the very early 20th century; simply because there was no way to see them until the invention of the electron microscope.

Viruses are peculiar creatures; believed to be on the borderline of living and non-living creatures; because in the external environment, they have been seen to 'exist' in crystalline form, and while inside a living system, they become active and reproduce.

Another peculiar distinction is that some viruses have RNA, instead of DNA as their genetic material. RNA, as a molecule, is far more unstable than DNA, hence DNA has been chosen as the genetic material of choice for all other living entities.

But that is not to say that these organisms are at a disadvantage; indeed these creatures are so potent that they have been known to cause the most lethal diseases, and time and again, give rise to more and more novel diseases which other living systems have found hard to tackle; take the *HIV virus*, the *Ebola* and *Marburg* Viruses, and of course, commonly the *Influenza Viruses* as testament to that.

RNA viruses generally have very high mutation rates as they lack DNA polymerases (enzymes which can find and fix mistakes when DNA is being replicated), and are therefore unable to conduct DNA repair of damaged genetic material. DNA viruses have considerably lower mutation rates due to the proof-reading ability of DNA polymerases within the host cell. Retroviruses (those viruses which have RNA as genetic material, but convert it to DNA once inside a living system, like HIV Virus) have a high mutation rate even though their DNA intermediate integrates into the host genome (and is thus subject to host DNA proofreading once integrated), because errors during reverse transcription are embedded into both strands of DNA prior to integration.

Although RNA usually mutates rapidly, recent work found that the SARS virus and related RNA viruses contain a gene that mutates very slowly. The gene in question has a complex three-dimensional structure which is hypothesized to provide a chemical function necessary for viral propagation, perhaps as a ribozyme. If so, most mutations would render it unfit for that purpose and would not propagate.

Seasonal Variations

Influenza viruses are the most common examples of viruses undergoing rapid mutations to alter their forms, and be able to cause outbreaks again and again.

Influenza reaches peak prevalence in winter, and because the Northern and Southern Hemispheres have winter at different times of the year, there are actually two different flu seasons each year. This is why the World Health Organization (assisted by the National Influenza Centers) makes recommendations for two different vaccine formulations every year; one for the Northern, and one for the Southern Hemisphere.

It is not clear why outbreaks of the flu occur seasonally rather than uniformly throughout the year. One possible explanation is that, because people are indoors more often during the winter, they are in close contact more often, and this promotes transmission from person to person. Another is that cold temperatures lead to drier air, which may dehydrate mucus, preventing the body from effectively expelling virus particles. The virus may also survive longer on exposed surfaces (doorknobs, countertops, etc.) in colder temperatures. Increased travel due to the Northern Hemisphere winter holiday season may also play a role.

A contributing factor is that aerosol transmission of the virus is highest in cold environments (less than 5°C) with low relative humidity. However, seasonal changes in infection rates also occur in tropical regions, and in some countries these peaks of infection are seen mainly during the rainy season. Seasonal changes in contact rates from school terms, which are a major factor in other childhood diseases such as measles and pertussis, may also play a role in the flu.

A combination of these small seasonal effects may be amplified by dynamical resonance with the endogenous disease cycles.

Epidemic and Pandemic Spread

As influenza is caused by a variety of species and strains of viruses, in any given year some strains can die out while others create epidemics, while yet another strain can cause a pandemic. An **epidemic** is defined as a consistent outbreak of a disease over a large geographic region, like a nation. A **pandemic** is defined as a consistent outbreak of a disease all over the world over a period of time.

Typically, in a year's normal two flu seasons (one per hemisphere), there are between three and five million cases of

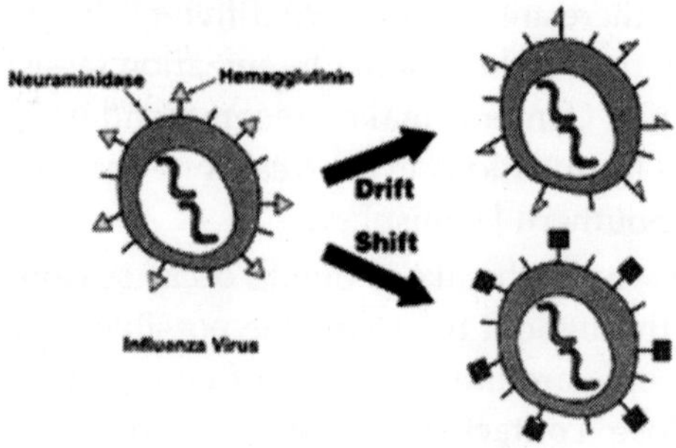

Figure a: Antigenic drift creates influenza viruses with slightly modified antigens, while antigenic shift generates viruses with entirely novel antigens.

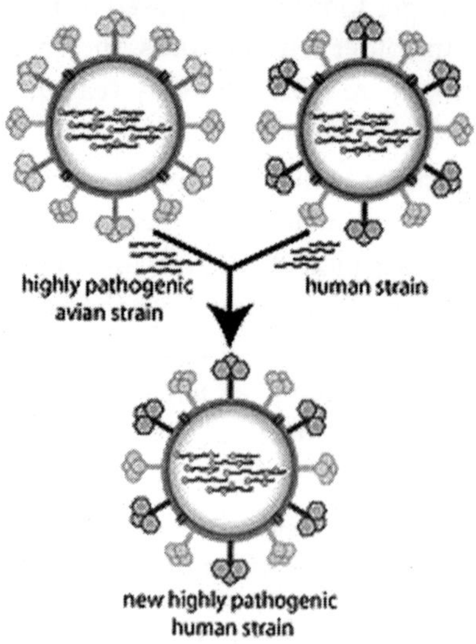

Figure b: Antigenic shift, or reassortment, can result in novel and highly pathogenic strains of human influenza

severe illness and up to 500,000 deaths worldwide, which by some definitions is a yearly influenza epidemic. Although the incidence of influenza can vary widely between years, approximately 36,000 deaths and more than 200,000 hospitalizations are directly associated with influenza every year in the United States.

Roughly three times per century, a pandemic occurs, which infects a large proportion of the world's population and can kill tens of millions of people.

New influenza viruses are constantly evolving by mutation or by reassortment. Mutations can cause small changes in the antigens (those molecules against which antibodies form) on the surface of the virus. This is called antigenic drift, which slowly creates an increasing variety of strains until one evolves that can infect people who are immune to the pre-existing strains. This new variant then replaces the older strains as it rapidly sweeps through the human population—often causing an epidemic.

However, since the strains produced by drift will still be reasonably similar to the older strains, some people will still be immune to them. In contrast, when influenza viruses reassort, they acquire completely new antigens—for example by reassortment between avian strains and human strains; this is called antigenic shift. If a human influenza virus is produced that has entirely new antigens, everybody will be susceptible, and the novel influenza will spread uncontrollably, causing a pandemic. In contrast to this model of pandemics based on antigenic drift and shift, an alternative approach has been proposed where the periodic pandemics are produced by interactions of a fixed set of viral strains with a human population with a constantly changing set of immunities to different viral strains.

Documented pandemics have occurred at intervals of 10 to 50 years since the 16th century including three in the last century. The most devastating of the last three, the 1918 "Spanish Influenza", caused the death of an estimated 20 to 40 million people.

The current widespread circulation of highly pathogenic influenza A (H5N1) virus in poultry and its occasional transmission to humans have raised concern that the world is moving closer to the next pandemic. While it is uncertain whether this particular virus will ever acquire the capacity for sustained human-to-human transmission, scientists agree that it is inevitable that another pandemic with an influenza virus will occur. The Severe Acute Respiratory Syndrome (SARS) that emerged in 2002 and 2003 affected 26 countries in less than five months and showed how fast an epidemic with a new pathogen can spread in modern society with air travel. This event also demonstrated the impact a public health crisis can have on a global economy.

Also, in spite of the disease being of a relatively mild nature, except in some risk groups, the disease has managed to travel far and wide in a short span of time. This could be attributable to the nature of the global economies today; like economic effects, the ripples of disease can also be felt all over.

It is seen that such diseases have traditionally been born in cultures where there is seen a close contact with animals. Wherever animals are reared and consumed in high quantities, the viruses circulating in them can gradually make a 'jump' and cross the 'species barrier' to infect newer species; this is a mechanism for their survival and propagation as well.

Importance of Surveillance to Detect and Respond to a Pandemic

Successful containment or control of pandemic influenza will rely on early recognition of sustained human-to-human transmission which requires a system for outbreak detection, rapid data collection, analysis, assessment and timely reporting. Early detection of the start of a pandemic is crucial to rapidly implement measures to stop the pandemic at its source and to prevent millions of deaths, social disruption and economic loss.

Modelling studies suggest that mass prophylaxis with antiviral drugs combined with other public health interventions such as movement restriction, social distancing, and vaccination may successfully contain an emerging pandemic. However, such an approach (i.e. rapid containment operation) would need to be implemented within the first few weeks that transmission of a pandemic virus began.

The goal of rapid containment is to delay, if not stop the pandemic. This will provide additional time for countries to implement public health actions, produce and distribute pandemic vaccines, and allow mobilization of international resources.

As part of national pandemic preparedness planning each country should prepare for enhanced surveillance to:

(i) Detect the emergence of the new disease

(ii) Characterize the disease (epidemiology, clinical manifestations, severity)

(iii) Monitor its evolution.

Benefits of Global Pandemic Influenza Surveillance

An influenza pandemic will affect every country. Standardized and coordinated international information sharing is crucial for crisis management at global and national levels. National authorities will need to know how the pandemic is evolving not only in their own country, but also in neighbouring countries and continents. Sharing of information at global level will be a benefit to all. The continual flow and aggregation of information provided by individual countries will contribute to the development of a global picture which:

- Will result in a rapid accumulation of critical clinical, epidemiological and virological data about the new disease
- Will allow health care providers and public health authorities to modify their strategies for case management, community mitigation, and health resource allocation
- Will disperse the workload among the first affected countries
- Will reduce the impact of inaccurate and unconfirmed rumours

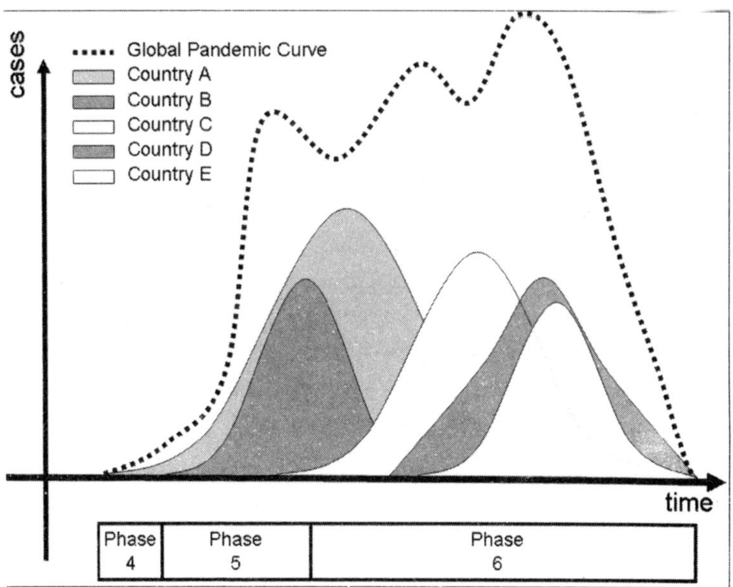

- Will enable WHO to serve as a credible and stabilizing source of information and guidance

Misinformation or lack of information at global or country level will inevitably result in delays in response, spread of damaging rumours, inadequate resource allocation, misdirected efforts, and ultimately, unnecessary loss of life.

The graph below highlights a global pandemic curve documented over a period of time: when the level of alertness progresses through stages four and five to reach the maximum possible alertness.

Phase Four

Human to human transmission of an animal or human-animal influenza reassortant virus able to sustain community-level outbreaks has been verified.

Phase Five

The virus has caused sustained community level outbreaks in two or more countries in one WHO Region.

Phase Six

The virus has caused sustained community level outbreaks in at least another country in another WHO Region in addition to the criteria defined in Phase five.

Sunaina Chaturvedi

Contents

Helpline Numbers in India

Emergency Contact Numbers in India

All India toll free H1N1 helpline, SWINE Flu helpline in Delhi, SWINE Flu helpline in Chennai, SWINE Flu helpline in Coimbatore, SWINE Flu helpline in Kolkata, SWINE Flu helpline in Hyderabad, SWINE Flu helpline in Mumbai, SWINE Flu helpline in Pune, SWINE Flu helpline in Bangalore, SWINE Flu helpline, full information helpline for Swine Flu

All India toll free H1N1 helpline: 1075 or 1800-11-4377

Delhi: Ram Manohar Lohia Hospital: 011-24525211, 23404328, 23365525

Deen Dayal Hospital: 011-2512 5259

Chennai: Communicable Diseases Hospital - 044-25912686.

Coimbatore Medical College Hospital - 09442012555

Kolkata: Infectious Diseases Hospital: 09433392182/ 09434009077

Hyderabad: AP Chest Diseases Hospital: 040-23814939

Mumbai: Kasturba Hospital: 022-23083901, 23083902, 23083903, 23083904

Pune: Dr Naidu Infectious Disease Hospital - 09923130909

Bangalore: Rajiv Gandhi Institute of Chest Diseases - 91-80-26632634

Lakeside Hospital: 80-5360823

Government Authorized Hospitals for Treatment of Swine Flu

Name of the Hospital	Address	Contact Numbers
City Hospital King Institute of Preventive Medicine (24/7 Service)	Guindy, Chennai–32	(044) 22501520, 22501521 & 22501522
Communicable Diseases Hospital	Thondiarpet, Chennai	(044) 25912686/87/ 88, 9444459543
Government General Hospital	Opp. Central Railway Station, Chennai – 03	(044) 25305000, 25305723, 25305721, 25330300
Naidu Hospital	Nr Le'Meridian, Raja Bahadur Mill, GPO, Pune-01	(020) 26058243
National Institute of Virology	20A Ambedkar Road, Pune - 11	(020) 26006290
Kolkata ID Hospital	57,Beliaghata, Beliaghata Road, Kolkata - 10	(033) 23701252
Coimbatore Government General Hospital	Near Railway Station, Trichy Road, Coimbatore-18	(0422) 2301393, 2301394, 2301395, 2301396
Hyderabad Govt. General and Chest Diseases Hospital	Erragadda, Hyderabad	(040) 23814939
Sir J J Hospital	J J Marg, Byculla, Mumbai-08	(022) 23735555, 23739031, 23760943, 23768400, 23731144/ 5555/23701393/1366

SDS Tuberculosis & Rajiv Gandhi Institute of Chest Diseases	Hosur Road, Hombegowda Nagar, Bangalore-29	(080) 26631923 Dr. Shivaraj - 99801-48780
Mumbai Haffkine Institute	Acharya Donde Marg, Parel, Mumbai-12	(022) 24160947, 24160961, 24160962
Government Medical College	Vandanam P O, Allapuzha-05	(0477) 2282015
Taluk Hospital	Railway Station Road, Alwaye, Ernakulam Kochi	(0484) 2624040 Sathyajit - 09847840051
Taluk Hospital	Perumbavoor PO, Ernakulam 542 Kochi	(0484) 2523138 Vipin - 09447305200
All India Institute of Medical Sciences (AIIMS)	Ansari Nagar, Aurobindo Marg Ring Road, New Delhi - 29	(011) 26594404, 26861698 Prof. R C Deka – 9868397464
National Institute for Communicable Diseases	22, Sham Nath Marg, New Delhi-54	(011) 23971272/060/ 344/524/449/326
Dr. Ram Manohar Lohia Hospital	Kharak Singh Marg, New Delhi-01	(011) 23741640, 23741649, 23741639 Dr. N K Chaturvedi – 9811101704
Vallabhai Patel Chest Institute	University Enclave, New Delhi-07	(011) 27667102, 27667441, 27667667, 27666182
Victoria Hospital	K R Market, Kalasipalayam, Bangalore-02	(080) 26703294 Dr. Gangadhar - 94480-49863
Government Medical College	Gandhi Nagar P O, Kottayam - 08	(0481) 2597311,2597312
Kasturba Gandhi Hospital	Arthur Road, N M Joshi Marg, Jacob Circle, Mumbai-11	(022) 23083901, 23092458, 23004512

CHAPTER 1

Introduction to Swine Flu

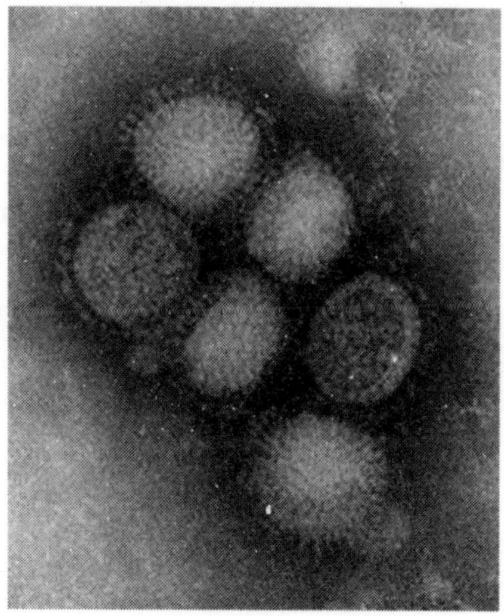

Swine influenza is an infection by any one of several types of Swine Influenza Virus. It is also called **H1N1 flu**, **swine flu**, **hog flu**, and **pig flu.** Normally, the **Swine Influenza Virus** (**SIV**) is any strain of the influenza family of viruses that is endemic in pigs.

As of 2009, the known SIV strains include Influenza C and the subtypes of influenza A known as H1N1, H1N2, H3N1, H3N2, and H2N3.

(right: Electron Micrograph of H1N1 Influenza Virus)

Swine Influenza Virus is common throughout pig populations worldwide. Transmission of the virus from pigs to humans is not common and does not always lead to human influenza, often resulting only in the production of antibodies in the blood.

If transmission does cause human influenza, it is called **zoonotic** swine flu (i.e. infection from animals). People with regular exposure to pigs are at increased risk of swine flu infection. The meat of an infected animal poses no risk of infection when properly cooked.

During the mid-20th century, identification of influenza subtypes became possible, allowing accurate diagnosis of transmission to humans. Since then, only 50 such transmissions have been confirmed. These strains of swine flu rarely pass from human to human. Symptoms of zoonotic swine flu in humans are similar to those of influenza and of influenza-like illness in general, namely chills, fever, sore throat, muscle pains, severe headache, coughing, weakness and general discomfort.

The **2009 flu pandemic** is a global outbreak of a new strain of influenza virus, officially named the **"new H1N1"**, first identified in April 2009, and commonly called **"Swine Flu."** This virus is actually not just a 'swine flu' virus, but is believed to be a mutation of four known strains of the influenza A virus, subtype H1N1: one endemic in (normally infecting) humans, one endemic in birds, and two endemic in pigs (swine).

Locus of Origin

Experts assume the virus "most likely" emerged from pigs in Asia, and was carried to North America by infected persons. Transmission of the new strain is human-to-human, with cooked pork products safe to eat as the virus cannot be transmitted by eating foods.

The outbreak began in Mexico, with evidence that Mexico was already in the midst of an epidemic for months before the outbreak was recognized. Soon after, its government closed down most of Mexico City's public and private offices and facilities to help contain the spread. In early June, as the virus spread globally, the World Health Organization (WHO) declared the outbreak to be a pandemic, but also noted that most illnesses were of "moderate severity."

The virus has since spread to the Southern Hemisphere which entered its winter flu season, and to many less developed countries with limited healthcare systems. Because the virus was spreading rapidly and many clinics were overwhelmed testing and treating patients, WHO stopped requiring countries to report all cases, but is still monitoring unusually large outbreaks.

The virus typically spreads from coughs and sneezes or by touching contaminated surfaces and then touching the nose or mouth. Symptoms, which can last up to a week, are similar to those of seasonal flu, and may include fever, sneezes, sore throat, coughs, headache, and muscle or joint pains.

The U.S. Centers for Disease Control and Prevention (CDC) notes that most cases worldwide have, so far, been mild and most hospitalizations and deaths have been of persons that also had underlying conditions such as asthma, diabetes, obesity, heart disease, or a weakened immune system. Then again, Dr Anne Schuchat from CDC thinks, "this is a virus that's capable of causing a spectrum of illness that includes severe complications and death". "It's very important we take this virus seriously".

As the virus spreads easily between people, through the air or surface contact, those who get the flu are recommended to stay home from school or work and avoid crowds to avoid spreading the infection further.

In an attempt to slow the spread of the illness, a number of countries, especially in Asia, have quarantined airline passengers with flu symptoms, while some are also pre-screening passengers. WHO does not expect to have a full vaccine before the end of 2009, and vaccines available sooner may be limited and given first to healthcare workers, pregnant women, and other higher risk groups. Two or three injections will be required for maximum immunity from both the swine flu and seasonal flu. There is also concern if the new virus mutates further, it could become more virulent and less susceptible to any new vaccine.

Debate on Nomenclature

Some authorities object to calling the flu outbreak "Swine Flu". U.S. Agriculture Secretary Tom Vilsack expressed concerns that this would lead to the misconception that pork is unsafe for consumption.

The CDC began referring to it as "Novel Influenza A (H1N1)". In the Netherlands, it was originally called "Pig Flu" and then called "Mexican Flu" by the National Health Institute and in the media. South Korea and Israel briefly considered calling it the

"Mexican Virus". Later, the South Korean press used "SI", short for "Swine Influenza". Taiwan suggested the names "H1N1 Flu" or "New Flu", which most local media now use. The World Organization for Animal Health proposed the name "North American Influenza". The European Commission adopted the term "Novel Flu Virus".

After initially opposing changing the name from "Swine Flu", the WHO announced they would refer to the new influenza virus as Influenza A (H1N1) or "Influenza A (H1N1) virus.

The outbreak was also called the "H1N1 Influenza"; "2009 H1N1 flu", or "Swine-origin Influenza".

In July 2009 WHO experts decided to call the virus "Pandemic H1N1/09 Virus" to distinguish it from the current seasonal H1N1 viruses in a way which was scientifically sound as well as to avoid some of the stigma associated with other options.

Yet, in spite of all specified nomenclatures, the Indian media and the Indian public refers to it as *Swine Flu*!

CHAPTER 2

The Flu: A Journey Back in Time

The name 'influenza' is said to have been given by Italians during the epidemic of 1743, which they ascribed to the malevolent influence of heavenly bodies or of inclement weather.

Annual influenza epidemics are estimated to affect 5–15% of the global population. Although most cases are mild, this still causes severe illness in 3–5 million people and around 250,000–500,000 deaths worldwide. In industrialized countries severe illness and deaths occur mainly in the high-risk populations of infants, the elderly and chronically ill patients.

In addition to these annual epidemics, Influenza A virus strains caused three major global epidemics during the 20th century: the Spanish flu in 1918, Asian flu in 1957 and Hong Kong flu in 1968-69. These pandemics were caused by strains of *Influenza A* virus that had undergone major genetic changes and for which the population did not possess significant immunity. The overall effects of these pandemics and epidemics are summarized in the table below.

The influenza virus has also caused several pandemic threats over the past century, including the pseudo-pandemic of 1947, the 1976 swine flu outbreak and the 1977 Russian flu, all caused by the H1N1 subtype.

20th century flu pandemics

Pandemic	Year	Influenza A virus subtype	People infected (approx)	Deaths (est.)	Case fatality rate
1918 flu pandemic	1918–19	H1N1	0.5 to 1 billion (near 50%)	20 to 50 million	>2.5%
Asian flu	1956–58	H2N2		2 million	<0.1% (?)
Hong Kong flu	1968–69	H3N2		1 million	<0.1%
Seasonal flu	Every year	mainly A/H3N2, A/H1N1, and B	5–15% (340 million-1 billion)	250,000–500,000 per year	<0.05%

The Seasonal Flu is not a pandemic, but listed to compare the several flu strains endemic in humans which produce seasonal flu with the rare new strain that results in a flu pandemic.

The world has been at an increased level of alert since the SARS epidemic in Southeast Asia (caused by the SARS coronavirus). The level of preparedness was further increased and sustained with the advent of the H5N1 bird flu outbreaks because of H5N1's high fatality rate, although the strains currently prevalent have limited human-to-human transmission (anthroponotic) capability, or epidemicity.

Case Study: The 1918 Spanish Flu Epidemic

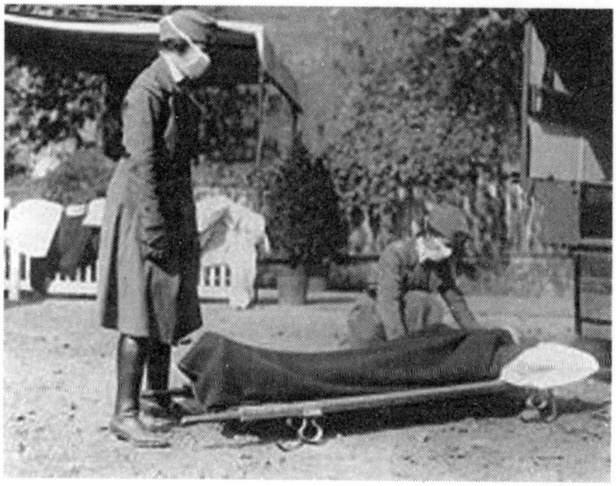

Image (right): Two American Red Cross nurses demonstrate treatment practices during the influenza pandemic of 1918.

The **1918 Spanish Flu Pandemic** was an influenza pandemic that spread to nearly every part of the world. It was caused by an unusually virulent and deadly *Influenza A Virus* strain of subtype *H1N1*. Historical and epidemiological data are inadequate to identify the geographic origin of the virus. Most of its victims were healthy young adults, in contrast to most influenza outbreaks which predominantly affect juvenile, elderly, or otherwise weakened patients.

The pandemic lasted from March 1918 to June 1920, spreading even to the Arctic and remote Pacific Islands. It is estimated that anywhere from 50 to 100 million people were killed worldwide. An estimated 500 million people, one third of the world's population (approximately 1.6 billion at the time), became infected.

Scientists have used tissue samples from frozen victims to reproduce the virus for study. Given the strain's extreme virulence there has been controversy regarding the wisdom of such research. Among the conclusions of this research is that the virus kills via a cytokine storm (overreaction of the body's immune system) which explains its unusually severe nature and the concentrated age profile of its victims. The strong immune systems of young adults ravaged the body, whereas the weaker immune systems of children and middle-aged adults caused fewer deaths.

The global mortality rate from the 1918/1919 pandemic is not known, but it is estimated that 10% to 20% of those who were infected died. With about a third of the world population infected, this case-fatality ratio means that 3% to 6% of the entire global population died. Influenza may have killed as many as 25 million in its first 25 weeks. Older estimates say it killed 40–50 million people while current estimates say 50 million to 100 million people worldwide were killed. This pandemic has been described as "the greatest medical holocaust in history" and may have killed more people than the Black Death.

This huge death toll was caused by an extremely high infection rate of up to 50% and the extreme severity of the symptoms, suspected to be caused by cytokine storms. Indeed, symptoms in 1918 were so unusual that initially influenza was misdiagnosed as dengue, cholera, or typhoid. One observer wrote, "One of the most striking of the complications was hemorrhage from mucous membranes, especially from the nose, stomach, and intestine. Bleeding from the ears and petechial hemorrhages in the skin also occurred." The majority of deaths were from bacterial pneumonia, a secondary infection caused by influenza, but the virus also killed people directly, causing massive hemorrhages and edema in the lungs.

The unusually severe disease killed between 2 and 20% of those infected, as opposed to the more usual flu epidemic mortality rate of 0.1%. Another unusual feature of this pandemic was that it mostly killed young adults, with 99% of pandemic influenza deaths occurring in people under 65, and more than half in young adults 20 to 40 years old. This is unusual since influenza is normally most deadly to the very young (under age 2) and the very old (over age 70), and may have been due to partial protection caused by exposure to a previous Russian flu pandemic of 1889.

Although the first cases of the disease were registered in the continental US and the rest of Europe long before getting to Spain, the 1918 Flu received its nickname "Spanish Flu" because Spain, a neutral country in WWI, had no special censorship for news against the disease and its consequences. Hence the most reliable news came from Spain, giving the false impression that Spain was the most—if not the only—affected zone.

A large factor of worldwide flu occurrence was increased travel. Modern transportation systems made it easier for soldiers, sailors, and civilian travelers to spread the disease quickly to communities worldwide.

Patterns of Fatality

The influenza strain was unusual in that this pandemic killed many young adults and otherwise healthy victims; typically influenza kills mostly weak individuals, such as infants (aged 0–2 years), the elderly, and the immuno-compromised. Older adults may have had some immunity from the earlier Russian flu pandemic of 1889. Another oddity was that the outbreak was widespread in the summer and autumn (in the Northern Hemisphere) when it is well documented that influenza is usually worse in winter.

In fast-progressing cases, mortality was primarily from pneumonia, by virus-induced pulmonary collapse. Slower-progressing cases featured secondary bacterial pneumonias, and there may have been neural (nervous system) involvement that led to mental disorders in some cases. Some deaths resulted from malnourishment and even animal attacks in overwhelmed communities.

Deadlier Second Time Around

The second wave of the 1918 pandemic was much deadlier than the first. During the first wave, which began in early March, the epidemic resembled typical flu epidemics. Those at the most risk were the sick and elderly, and younger, healthier people recovered easily. But in August, when the second wave began in France, Sierra Leone and the United States, the virus had mutated to a much more deadly form. This has been attributed to the circumstances of the First World War.

In civilian life evolutionary pressures favour a mild strain: those who get really sick stay at home, but those mildly ill continue with their lives, go to work and go shopping, preferentially spreading the mild strain. In the trenches the evolutionary pressures were reversed: soldiers with a mild strain remained where they were, while the severely ill were sent on crowded trains to crowded field hospitals, spreading the deadlier virus. So the second wave began and flu quickly spread around the world again. It was the same flu, in that those who recovered from first-wave infections were immune, but it was far more deadly, and the most vulnerable people were those like the soldiers in the trenches - young, otherwise healthy, adults. Consequently, during modern pandemics, health officials pay attention when the virus reaches places with social upheaval, looking for deadlier strains of the virus.

Devastated Communities

Even in areas where mortality was low, so many people were incapacitated that much of everyday life stopped. Some communities closed all stores or required customers to leave their orders outside the store. There were many reports of places where the health-care workers could not tend the sick nor the grave-diggers bury the dead because they too were ill. Mass graves were dug by steam shovel and bodies buried without coffins in many places. Several Pacific Island territories were particularly hard-hit.

The pandemic reached them from New Zealand, which was too slow to implement measures to prevent ships carrying the flu from leaving its ports. From New Zealand, the flu reached Tonga (killing 8% of the population), Nauru (16%) and Fiji (5%, 9000 people). Worst affected was Western Samoa, a territory then under New Zealand military administration. A crippling 90% of the population was infected; 30% of adult men, 22% of adult women and 10% of children were killed. By contrast, the flu was kept away from American Samoa by a commander who imposed a blockade. The mortality rate in New Zealand itself was 5%.

Less Affected Areas

In Japan, 257,363 deaths were attributed to influenza by July 1919, giving an estimated 0.425% mortality rate, much lower than nearly all other Asian countries for which data are available. The Japanese government severely restricted maritime travel to and from the home islands when the pandemic struck.

In the Pacific, American Samoa and the French colony of New Caledonia also succeeded in preventing even a single death from influenza through effective quarantines. In Australia, nearly 12,000 perished.

End of the Pandemic

After the lethal second wave struck in the autumn of 1918, the disease died down abruptly. New cases almost dropped to nothing after the peak in the second wave. In Philadelphia for example, 4,597 people died in the week ending October 16, but by November 11 influenza had almost disappeared from the city. One explanation for the rapid decline of the lethality of the disease is that doctors simply got better at preventing and treating the pneumonia which developed after the victims had contracted the virus. Another theory holds that the 1918 virus mutated extremely rapidly to a less lethal strain. This is a common occurrence with influenza viruses: there is a general tendency for pathogenic viruses to become less lethal as time goes by, providing more living hosts. According to this theory, this happened very quickly for the 1918 virus.

The majority of fatalities, in both World War I and in the Spanish Flu epidemic, were young adults. The deaths caused by the flu may have been overlooked due to the large numbers of deaths of young men in the war or as a result of injuries. When people read the obituaries of the era, they saw the war or post-war deaths and the deaths from the influenza side by side. In particular in Europe, where the war's toll was extremely high, the flu may not have had a great, separate, psychological impact, or may have seemed a mere "extension" of the war's tragedies.

The duration of the pandemic and the war could also play a role: the disease would usually only affect a certain area for a month before leaving, while the war, which most expected to end quickly, had lasted for four years by the time the pandemic struck. This left little time for the disease to have a significant impact on the economy.

During this time period pandemic outbreaks were not uncommon: typhoid, yellow fever, diphtheria, and cholera all occurred near the same time period. These outbreaks probably lessened the significance of the influenza pandemic for the public.

Research on the Emergence of such a Virulent Strain

One theory is that the virus strain originated at Fort Riley, Kansas, by two genetic mechanisms – *antigenic drift* and *antigenic shift* – in viruses in poultry and swine which the fort bred for food; the soldiers were then sent from there to different places around the world, where they spread the disease.

However, evidence from a recent reconstruction of the virus suggests that it jumped directly from birds to humans, without traveling through swine. This suggestion is however controversial, and other research suggests that the strain originated in a mammalian species.

An effort to recreate the 1918 flu strain (a subtype of avian strain H1N1) was a collaboration among the Armed Forces Institute of Pathology, Southeast Poultry Research Laboratory and Mount Sinai School of Medicine in New York; the effort resulted in the announcement (on October 5, 2005) that the group had successfully determined the virus's genetic sequence, using historic tissue samples recovered by pathologist Johan Hultin from a female flu victim buried in the Alaskan permafrost and samples preserved from American soldiers.

On January 18, 2007, Kobasa et al. reported that monkeys (*Macaca fascicularis*) infected with the recreated strain exhibited classic symptoms of the 1918 pandemic and died from a cytokine storm – an overreaction of the immune system. This may explain why the 1918 flu had its surprising effect on younger, healthier people, as a person with a stronger immune system would potentially have a stronger overreaction.

On September 16, 2008, the body of a Yorkshireman, Sir Mark Sykes was exhumed to study the RNA of the Spanish flu virus in efforts to understand the genetic structure of modern H5N1 bird flu. Sykes had been buried in 1919 in a lead coffin which scientists hope will have helped preserve the virus.

In December, 2008 research by Yoshihiro Kawaoka of University of Wisconsin linked the presence of three specific genes (termed PA, PB1, and PB2) and a nucleoprotein derived from 1918 flu samples to the ability of the flu virus to invade the lungs and cause pneumonia. The combination triggered similar symptoms in animal testing.

Case: Swine Flu

1976 Swine Flu Outbreak

The **1976 Swine Flu Outbreak**, also known as the **Swine Flu Fiasco**, or the **Swine Flu Debacle**, was a strain of H1N1 Influenza Virus that appeared in 1976. Infections were only detected from January 19 to February 9, and were not found outside Fort Dix. Even though there were rapid vaccinations against the virus, side-effects from the vaccine caused 25 deaths.

On February 15, 1976, an army recruit at Fort Dix said he felt tired and weak. He died the next day and four of his fellow soldiers were later hospitalized. Two weeks after his death, health officials announced that *Swine Flu* was the cause of death and that this strain of flu appeared to be closely related to the strain involved in the 1918 flu pandemic. Alarmed public health officials decided that action must be taken to head off another major pandemic, and they urged the then President Gerald Ford that every person in the U.S. be vaccinated for the disease. The vaccination program was plagued by delays and public relations problems, but about 24% of the population had been vaccinated by the time the program was canceled. Only one person, the Fort Dix army recruit, died from the flu.

There were reports of Guillain-Barré syndrome, a paralyzing neuromuscular disorder, affecting some people who had received swine flu immunizations. This syndrome is a rare side effect of modern influenza vaccines, with an incidence of about one case per million vaccinations.

Overall, about 500 cases of Guillain-Barré syndrome (GBS), resulting in death from severe pulmonary complications for 25 people, were probably caused by an immuno-pathological reaction to the 1976 vaccine. Other influenza vaccines have not been linked to Guillain-Barré syndrome, though caution is advised for certain individuals, particularly those with a history of GBS.

Etymology

Swine influenza was first proposed to be a disease related to human influenza during the 1918 flu pandemic, when pigs became sick at the same time as humans. The first identification of an influenza virus as a cause of disease in pigs occurred about ten years later, in 1930. For the following 60 years, swine influenza strains were almost exclusively H1N1. Then, between 1997 and 2002, new strains of three different subtypes and five different genotypes emerged as causes of influenza among pigs in North America. In 1997-98, H3N2 strains emerged. These strains, which include genes derived by reassortment from human, swine and avian viruses, have become a major cause of swine influenza in North America. Reassortment between H1N1 and H3N2 produced H1N2. In 1999 in Canada, a strain of H4N6 crossed the species barrier from birds to pigs, but was contained on a single farm.

Swine flu has been reported numerous times as a zoonosis in humans, usually with limited distribution, rarely with a widespread distribution.

The H1N1 form of swine flu is one of the descendants of the strain that caused the 1918 flu pandemic. As well as persisting in pigs, the descendants of the 1918 virus have also circulated in humans through the 20th century, contributing to the normal seasonal epidemics of influenza.

However, direct transmission from pigs to humans is rare, with only 12 cases in the U.S. since 2005. Nevertheless, the retention of influenza strains in pigs after these strains have disappeared from the human population might make pigs a reservoir where influenza viruses could persist, later emerging to reinfect humans once human immunity to these strains has waned.

This new strain appeared to be closely related to the strain involved in the 1918 flu pandemic. Moreover, the ensuing increased surveillance uncovered another strain in circulation in the U.S.: Influenza A H3N2 spread simultaneously, also caused illness, and persisted until March. Alarmed public health officials decided action must be taken to head off another major pandemic.

1998 US Outbreak in Swine

In 1998, swine flu was found in pigs in four U.S. states. Within a year, it had spread through pig populations across the United States. Scientists found that this virus had originated in pigs as a recombinant form of flu strains from birds and humans. This outbreak confirmed that pigs can serve as a crucible where novel influenza viruses emerge as a result of the reassortment of genes from different strains.

2007 Phillippine Outbreak in Swine

On August 20, 2007, the Department of Agriculture officers investigated the outbreak (epizootic) of swine flu in Nueva Ecija and Central Luzon, Philippines. The mortality rate is less than 10% for swine flu, unless there are complications. On July 27, 2007, the Philippine National Meat Inspection Service (NMIS) raised a hog cholera *"red alert"* warning over Metro Manila and five regions of Luzon after the disease spread to backyard pig farms in Bulacan and Pampanga, even if these tested negative for the swine flu virus.

2009 Outbreak in Humans

The H1N1 viral strain implicated in the 2009 flu pandemic among humans often is called "swine flu" because initial testing showed many of the genes in the virus were similar to influenza viruses normally occurring in North American swine. But further research has shown that the outbreak is due to a new strain of H1N1 not previously reported in pigs.

In late April, Margaret Chan, the World Health Organization's director-general, declared a "public health emergency of international concern" under the rules of the WHO's new International Health Regulations when the first cases of the H1N1 virus were reported in the United States. Following the outbreak, on May 2, 2009, it was reported in pigs at a farm in Alberta, Canada, with a link to the outbreak in Mexico. The pigs are suspected to have caught this new strain of virus from a farm worker who recently returned from Mexico and had shown symptoms of an influenza-like illness. These are probable cases, pending confirmation by laboratory testing.

The new strain was initially described as an apparent reassortment of at least four strains of influenza A virus subtype H1N1, including one strain endemic in humans, one endemic in birds, and two endemic in swine. Subsequent analysis suggested it was a reassortment of just two strains, both found in swine.

Although initial reports identified the new strain as swine influenza (i.e. a zoonosis originating in swine), its origin is unknown. Several countries took precautionary measures to reduce the chances for a global pandemic of the disease. This particular Swine Flu has been compared to other similar types of influenzas in terms of mortality: *"in the US it appears that for every 1000 people who get infected, about 40 people need admission to hospital and about one person dies"*.

There were fears that swine flu would become a major global pandemic in the winter months, with many countries planning major vaccination campaigns. Since then, the situation has worsened; the WHO has declared it as a 'pandemic', and there are numerous cases that are being reported on a day-to-day basis now.

Initial Outbreaks

It is not known where the virus originated. Analysis has suggested that the H1N1 strain responsible for the current outbreak first evolved around September 2008 and circulated in the human population for several months before the first cases were identified as being due to a new strain.

Mexico

The virus was first reported in two U.S. children in March, but health officials have said that it apparently infected people as early as last January in Mexico. The outbreak was first detected in Mexico City on March 18, 2009, and health officials later confirmed an outbreak in Veracruz State in February. Immediately after the outbreak was officially announced, Mexico requested material support from the U.S., sending samples to the U.S. and Canada for testing.

Scientists tried to understand why there were so many deaths in Mexico while infections in the United States and Canada were relatively mild. Some experts now assume that Mexico already had hundreds of thousands, and possibly millions, of cases before the outbreak was officially recognized, and were therefore in the midst of a "silent epidemic."

As a result, Mexico was reporting only the most serious cases, and led a CDC expert to speculate at the time, "We may just be looking at the tip of the iceberg, which would give you a skewed initial estimate of the case fatality rate.

United States

The new strain was first diagnosed in two children, neither of whom had been in contact with pigs, by the CDC, first on April 14, 2009 in San Diego County, California and a few days later in nearby Imperial County, California (it was not identified as a new strain in Mexico until 24 April).

Estimates of Total Cases

On July 24, 2009, Keiji Fukuda, WHO's Assistant Director-General for Health Security and Environment said the pandemic was still in its early stages globally and two billion infections over the course of the pandemic was "a reasonable ballpark to be looking at."

On the same day, the Anne Schuchat, Director of the U.S. CDC's National Center for Immunization and Respiratory Diseases, estimated that without a swine flu vaccine, current trends suggest 12% to 24% of Americans might get swine flu this fall and winter. But if large enough numbers of people get the vaccine before the next waves of the pandemic sweep the nation it would "put a dent in the pandemic," she said.

As for the current totals, in early July WHO officials gave up trying to count the number of cases, saying the best they can do is estimate the spread of the "unstoppable" virus.

In late June, the CDC estimated that 1 million Americans had so far contracted the flu. By comparison, an estimated 15 million to 60 million Americans are infected with the seasonal flu each year, leading to roughly 36,000 deaths. According to the CDC, however, only about one in 20 cases was being officially reported in the U.S. in late May. In the U.K., some experts thought the number of cases was potentially 300 times more than the earlier published estimates, warning that case estimates by the U.K. and other governments were "meaningless" and hiding its true extent. There were also estimates that Japan may have had approximately 30,000 cases by late May.

CHAPTER 3

Pathology of the Disease

The H1N1 virus is a novel strain of influenza. Existing vaccines against seasonal flu provide no protection, and there is no vaccine for this strain. A study at the U.S. Centers for Disease Control and Prevention published in May 2009 found that children had no preexisting immunity to the new strain but that adults, particularly those over 60, had some degree of immunity. Children showed no cross-reactive antibody reaction to the new strain, adults aged 18 to 64 had 6-9%, and older adults 33%.

It was also determined that the strain contained genes from four different flu viruses: *North American Swine Influenza, North American Avian Influenza, Human Influenza,* and two *Swine Influenza* viruses typically found in Asia and Europe.

Further analysis showed that several of the proteins of the virus are most similar to strains that cause mild symptoms in humans. Leading virologist Wendy Barclay has suggested that the initial indications are that the virus was unlikely to cause severe symptoms for most people. Scientists in Winnipeg completed the first full genetic sequencing of the virus on 6 May, 2009.

Origin of the Virus

On June 23, the *New York Times* reported that U.S. Federal agriculture officials now believed that the new swine flu pandemic most likely arose in Asia and travelled to North America in a human, but there was no way to prove this theory. They stated that there is no evidence that this new virus, which combines Eurasian and North American genes, has ever circulated in North American pigs, "while there is tantalizing evidence that a closely related 'sister virus' has circulated in Asia."

In early June 2009, using computational methods developed over the last ten years at Oxford, Dr Oliver Pybus of Oxford University's Department of Zoology and his team attempted to reconstruct the origins and timescale of the 2009 flu pandemic. He claims "Our results show that this strain has been circulating among pigs, possibly among multiple continents, for many years prior to its transmission to humans."

The research team that worked on this report also believe that it was "derived from several viruses circulating in swine," and that the initial transmission to humans occurred several months before recognition of the outbreak. The team concluded that "despite widespread influenza surveillance in humans, the lack of systematic swine surveillance allowed for the undetected persistence and evolution of this potentially pandemic strain for many years."

According to the researchers, movement of live pigs between Eurasia and North America "seems to have facilitated the mixing of diverse swine influenza viruses, leading to the multiple reassortment events associated with the genesis of the (new H1N1) strain." They also stated that this new pandemic "provides further evidence of the role of domestic pigs in the ecosystem of influenza A." Some experts also suspect that a leading cause of the new virus outbreak is insufficient surveillance by the pork industry and the fact that "animal husbandry now more closely resembles the petrochemical industry than the happy family farm."

Virus Characteristics

The Swine Flu Virus is a typical animal virus, with a membranous envelope covering the protein capsid. The genetic material for the virus is a single stranded RNA.

St. of the Influenza Virion. The **Hemagglutinin (HA)** and **Neuraminidase (NA)** proteins are shown on the surface of the particle. The viral **RNAs** that make up the genome are shown as

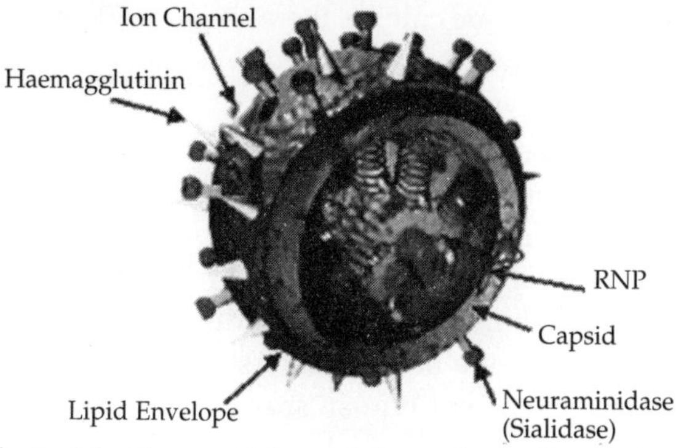

red coils inside the particle and bound to **ribonucleoproteins (RNPs).**

Influenza A

Swine influenza is known to be caused by influenza A subtypes H1N1, H1N2, H3N1, H3N2, and H2N3. In pigs, three Influenza A virus subtypes (H1N1, H3N2, and H1N2) are the most common strains worldwide.

In the United States, the H1N1 subtype was exclusively prevalent among swine populations before 1998; however, since late August 1998, H3N2 subtypes have been isolated from pigs. As of 2004, H3N2 virus isolates in US swine and turkey stocks were triple reassortments, containing genes from human (HA, NA, and PB1), swine (NS, NP, and M), and avian (PB2 and PA) lineages.

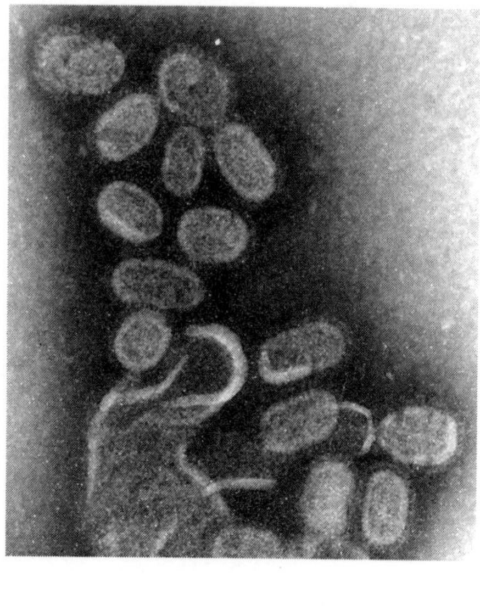

The physical structure of all Influenza A viruses is similar. The virions or virus particles are enveloped and can be either spherical or filamentous in form. In clinical isolates that have undergone limited passages in eggs or tissue culture, there are more filamentous than spherical particles, whereas passaged laboratory strains consist mainly of spherical virions.

Of the three genera of Influenza viruses that cause human flu, two also cause influenza in pigs, with Influenza A being common in pigs and Influenza C being rare. Influenza B has not been reported in pigs. Within Influenza A and Influenza C, the strains found in pigs and humans are largely distinct, although due to reassortment there have been transfers of genes among strains crossing swine, avian, and human species boundaries.

Influenza C

Influenza C viruses infect both humans and pigs, but do not infect birds. Transmission between pigs and humans has occurred in the past. For example, Influenza C caused small outbreaks of a mild form of influenza amongst children in Japan and California. Due to its limited host range and the lack of genetic diversity in the Influenza C Virus, this form of influenza does not cause pandemics in humans.

Virulence

The CDC has noted that most infections continue to be mild—similar to seasonal flu—and recovery is extremely quick.

Some experts point out that the deaths so far are "a tiny fraction" of people who die every year from seasonal flu - with barely a public murmur." One doctor said that "when there's something that's new and unknown, it scares people."

Some medical journalists suggest that the news media may be overreacting to the new virus and have not compared its virulence with that of the regular "seasonal" flu.

It has now been documented in most deaths that the death was caused not directly due to the flu, but also due to an already existing condition, like diabetes, asthma, hypertension and so on coupled with a flu-like illness which would become too much for the body to cope with.

Mutation Potential

On May 22, 2009, WHO chief Dr. Margaret Chan said that the virus must be closely monitored in the southern hemisphere, as it could mix with ordinary seasonal influenza and change in unpredictable ways. "In cases where the H1N1 virus is widespread and circulating within the general community, countries must expect to see more cases of severe and fatal infections," she said.

Experts writing in the July *New England Journal of Medicine* note that historically, pandemic viruses have evolved between seasons, and the current strain may become more severe or transmissible in the coming months. They therefore stress that "international cooperation will be crucial" to engage in proper surveillance to help monitor changes in the virus's behavior, which will aid in both "vaccine targeting" and interpreting illness patterns in the fall of 2009.

Other experts are also concerned that the new virus strain could mutate over the coming months. Guan Yi, a leading virologist from the University of Hong Kong, for instance, described the new H1N1 influenza virus as "very unstable", meaning it could mix and swap genetic material when exposed to other viruses. During an interview he said "Both H1N1 and H5N1 are unstable so the chances of them exchanging genetic material are higher, whereas a stable (seasonal flu) virus is less likely to take on genetic material."

The H5N1 virus is mostly limited to birds, but in rare cases when it infects humans it has a mortality rate of between 60% to 70%. Experts worry about the emergence of a hybrid of the more virulent Asian-lineage HPAI (highly pathogenic avian influenza) A/H5N1 strain (media labeled "bird flu") with more human-transmissible Influenza A strains such as this novel 2009 swine-origin A/H1N1 strain (media labeled "swine flu"), especially since the H5N1 strain is and has been for years endemic in birds in countries like China, Indonesia, Vietnam and Egypt.

Nor had federal health officials in the U.S. dismissed the possibility that the worst was yet to come. "Far from it," Ann

Schuchat of the CDC says, noting that the horrific 1918 flu epidemic, which killed hundreds of thousands in the United States alone, was preceded by a mild "herald" wave of cases in the spring, followed by devastating waves of illness in the autumn.

As of late July, U.S. health officials said that the swine flu "isn't yet mutating to become more dangerous," but they are closely tracking that as the virus continues to circle the globe.

Modes of Transmission

People who contract influenza are most infective between the second and third days after infection and infectivity lasts for around ten days. Children are much more infectious than adults and shed virus from just before they develop symptoms until two weeks after infection. The transmission of influenza can be modeled mathematically, which helps predict how the virus will spread in a population.

Influenza can be spread in three main ways:

- By direct transmission when an infected person sneezes mucus into the eyes, nose or mouth of another person
- Through people inhaling the aerosols produced by infected people coughing, sneezing and spitting
- Through hand-to-mouth transmission from either contaminated surfaces or direct personal contact, such as a hand-shake

The relative importance of these three modes of transmission is unclear, and they may all contribute to the spread of the virus. In the airborne route, the droplets that are small enough for people to inhale are 0.5 to 5 μm in diameter and inhaling just one droplet might be enough to cause an infection. Although a single sneeze releases up to 40,000 droplets, most of these droplets are quite large and will quickly settle out of the air. How long influenza survives in airborne droplets seems to be influenced by the levels of humidity and UV radiation: with low humidity and a lack of sunlight in winter probably aiding its survival.

As the influenza virus can persist outside of the body, it can also be transmitted by contaminated surfaces such as banknotes doorknobs, light switches and other household items. The length of time the virus will persist on a surface varies, with the virus surviving for one to two days on hard, non-porous surfaces such as plastic or metal, for about fifteen minutes from dry paper tissues, and only five minutes on skin. However, if the virus is present in mucus, this can protect it for longer periods. Avian influenza viruses can survive indefinitely when frozen. They are inactivated by heating to 56°C (133°F) for a minimum of 60 minutes, as well as by acids (at pH <2).

Transmission between Pigs

Influenza is quite common in pigs, with about half of breeding pigs having been exposed to the virus in the US. Antibodies to the virus are also common in pigs in other countries.

The main route of transmission is through direct contact between infected and uninfected animals. These close contacts are particularly common during animal transport. Intensive farming may also increase the risk of transmission, as the pigs are raised in very close proximity to each other.

The direct transfer of the virus probably occurs either by pigs touching noses, or through dried mucus. Airborne transmission through the aerosols produced by pigs coughing or sneezing is also an important means of infection.

The virus usually spreads quickly through a herd, infecting all the pigs within just a few days. Transmission may also occur through wild animals, such as wild boar, which can spread the disease between farms.

Transmission to Humans

The virus spreads by aerosol droplets, meaning that secretions from an infected person can be spread into the air by coughing or sneezing. It is the close contact with an ill person that causes the disease to spread. And a person may be contagious for 24 hours before any symptoms occur.

People who work with poultry and swine, especially people with intense exposures, are at increased risk of zoonotic infection with influenza virus endemic in these animals, and constitute a population of human hosts in which zoonosis and reassortment can co-occur.

Vaccination of these workers against influenza and surveillance for new influenza strains among this population may therefore be an important public health measure.

Other professions at particular risk of infection are veterinarians and meat processing workers, although the risk of infection for both of these groups is lower than that of farm workers.

Interaction with Avian H5N1 in Pigs

Pigs are unusual as they can be infected with influenza strains that usually infect three different species: pigs, birds and humans. This makes pigs a host where influenza viruses might exchange genes, producing new and dangerous strains.

Avian Influenza Virus H3N2 is endemic in pigs in China and has been detected in pigs in Vietnam, increasing fears of the emergence of new variant strains. H3N2 evolved from by antigenic shift. In August 2004, researchers in China found H5N1 in pigs.

Pathophysiology

The mechanisms by which influenza infection causes symptoms in humans have been studied intensively. Consequently, knowing which genes are carried by a particular strain can help predict how well it will infect humans and how severe this infection will be; that is, predict the strain's pathophysiology).

The virus usually enters via the respiratory tract, with its infectious dose (the minimum number of particlles required to create an infection) being very small; at 3 virion particles only!

Part of the process that allows influenza viruses to invade cells is the cleavage of the viral hemagglutinin protein by any one of several human proteases (protein degrading enzymes). In mild and avirulent viruses, the structure of the hemagglutinin means that it can only be cleaved by proteases found in the throat and lungs, so these viruses cannot infect other tissues. However, in highly virulent strains, such as H5N1, the hemagglutinin can be cleaved by a wide variety of proteases, allowing the virus to spread throughout the body.

The viral hemagglutinin protein is responsible for determining both which species a strain can infect and where in the human respiratory tract a strain of influenza will bind. Strains that are easily transmitted between people have hemagglutinin proteins that bind to receptors in the upper part of the respiratory tract, such as in the nose, throat and mouth. In contrast, the highly-lethal H5N1 strain binds to receptors that are mostly found deep in the lungs. This difference in the site of infection may be part of the reason why the H5N1 strain causes severe viral pneumonia in the lungs, but is not easily transmitted by people coughing and sneezing.

The neuraminidase is responsible for decreasing the viscosity off the lining of the mucous membrane in the respiratory tract to expose receptors for binding. This particular step is manifested by the running nose seen as the most obvious flu symptom.

Common symptoms of the flu such as fever, headaches, and fatigue are the result of the huge amounts of proinflammatory cytokines and chemokines (such as interferon or tumor necrosis factor) produced from influenza-infected cells.

In contrast to the *Rhinovirus* that causes the common cold, influenza does cause tissue damage, so symptoms are not entirely due to the inflammatory response. This massive immune response might produce a life-threatening cytokine storm. This effect has been proposed to be the cause of the unusual lethality of both the H5N1 avian influenza, and the 1918 pandemic strain. However, another possibility is that these large amounts of cytokines are just a result of the massive levels of viral replication produced by these strains, and the immune response does not itself contribute to the disease.

The cells which are damaged are shed off after an infection which exposes the trachea and the bronchi of the lungs. This, in turn, makes the respiraoty tract highly susceptible to secondary infection by bacteria.

Symptoms

The incubation period is about 1-3 days, following which there is the onset of symptoms.

In Swine

The main symptoms in infected pigs include:

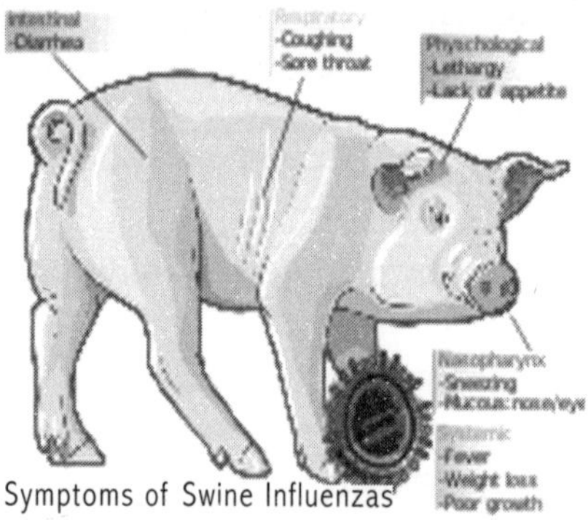

Symptoms of Swine Influenzas

- Fever
- Lethargy
- Sneezing
- Coughing
- Breathing Difficulty
- Decreased appetite
- In some cases, abortion

Although mortality is usually low (around 1-4%), the virus can produce weight loss and poor growth, causing economic loss to farmers. Infected pigs can lose up to 12 pounds of body weight over a 3 to 4 week period.

In Humans

Despite the apparently low numbers of infections, the true rate of infection may be higher, since most cases only cause a very mild disease, and will probably never be reported or diagnosed.

According to the Centers for Disease Control and Prevention (CDC), in humans the symptoms of the 2009 "swine flu" H1N1 virus are similar to those of influenza and of influenza-like illness in general.

The 2009 H1N1 virus is not zoonotic swine flu, as it is not transmitted from pigs to humans, but from person to person.

The main symptoms include:

- Fever (body temperature of 38 degrees and above)
- Cough
- Sore throat
- Running nose
- Body aches
- Headache
- Joint pain
- Chills
- Fatigue
- Diarrhea
- Vomiting
- Loss of appetite

Symptoms of Swine Flu

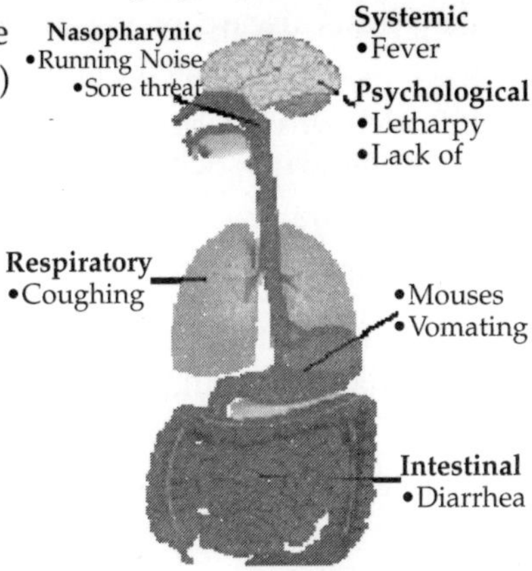

Since these symptoms are not specific to swine flu, a differential diagnosis of *probable* swine flu requires not only symptoms but also a high likelihood of swine flu due to the person's recent history.

For example, during the 2009 swine flu outbreak in the United States, CDC has advised physicians to consider swine influenza infection in the differential diagnosis of patients with acute febrile respiratory illness who have either been in contact with persons with confirmed swine flu, or who were in one of the five U.S. states that have reported swine flu cases or in Mexico during the 7 days preceding their illness onset. A diagnosis of *confirmed* swine flu requires laboratory testing of a respiratory sample (a simple nose and throat swab).

The most common cause of death is respiratory failure, other causes of death are pneumonia (leading to sepsis), high fever (leading to neurological problems), dehydration (from excessive vomiting and diarrhea) and electrolyte imbalance. Fatalities are more likely in young children and the elderly.

A study concluded on May 5, published in the New England Journal of Medicine, found that 94% of confirmed patients had fever and 92% had cough. People at higher risk of serious complications included people age 65 years and older, children younger than 5 years old, pregnant women, and people of any age with underlying medical conditions, such as asthma, diabetes, obesity, heart disease, or a weakened immune system (e.g., taking immunosuppressive medications or infected with HIV). According to the CDC, more than 70% of hospitalizations in the U.S. have been people with such underlying conditions.

Most Cases Mild

Evidence mounted through May 2009 that the symptoms were milder than health officials initially feared. Most of the confirmed cases in had been mild and there had been few deaths from the virus.

Similarly, Japan has reported 1,048, mostly mild flu cases, and no deaths, with the government reopening schools as of May 23, stating that the "virus should be considered more like a seasonal flu. In Mexico, where the outbreak began in April, Mexico City officials lowered their swine flu alert level as no new cases had been reported for a week.

The virus is now rapidly spreading across various parts in India with over 1200 cases confirmed. Again, most infections have been mild, although lax in treatment and other existing medical conditions have taken the death toll to 23 by August 14th 2009.

Symptoms that May Require Medical Attention

Certain symptoms may require emergency medical attention.

Symptoms in Children

- Signs of respiratory distress
- Blue lips and skin
- Dehydration
- Rapid breathing
- Excessive sleeping
- Seizures and
- Significant irritability including a lack of desire to be held

Symptoms in Adults

- Shortness of breath
- Pain in the chest or abdomen
- Sudden dizziness or confusion

In both children and adults, persistent vomiting or the return of flu-like symptoms that include a fever and cough may require medical attention.

Underlying Conditions May Worsen Symptoms

WHO reported that almost one-half of the patients hospitalized in the United States had underlying conditions A WHO report stated that among 30 patients hospitalized in California, 64 percent had underlying conditions and two of five pregnant women developed complications, including spontaneous abortion and premature rupture of membranes. And on June 5, health officials in six states that reported deaths from swine flu said that all six patients had been diagnosed with other health problems.

However, doctors in New York suggested that people with underlying conditions who had flu symptoms should consult their doctors first, for there is a strong possibility that if they do not already have the disease, they might catch it from the hospital waiting room.

In case patients are:

- Already having a serious existing illness that weakens the immune system, such as cancer
- Treatment, such as a transplant which leads to immunosuppression
- Expecting mothers
- Chronic (long-term) lung disease
- Chronic heart disease
- Chronic kidney disease
- Chronic liver disease
- Chronic neurological disease (neurological disorders include motor neurone disease, multiple sclerosis and Parkinson's disease),
- Diabetes Mellitus.
- Those who have had drug treatment for asthma within the past three years
- People aged 65 and older
- Young children under five
- Unwell children under one year of age

- Suddenly experiencing worst conditions
- Feeling their condition is not getting better after seven days (five for a child)

Pneumonia

Influenza infection can cause pneumonia leading to death. This is typically described as either viral pneumonia, which has a rapid onset, often within one day after infection, or bacterial pneumonia, which often begins a week after infection after symptoms have begun to subside.

Viral pneumonia has sometimes been attributed to "cytokine storm", in which an overly active immune response damages the lungs. Reports of deaths among healthy young people during the first weeks of the 2009 flu pandemic were attributed to this cause.

Bacterial pneumonia is a secondary infection resulting from a weakened ability to clear common bacteria from the lower lungs, combined with reduced alveolar macrophage activity which makes it more difficult for the body to fight infection.

Bacteria that cause pneumonia include *Pneumococcus, Staphylococcus,* and *Hemophilus influenzae.* Bacterial pneumonia has been credited for a large proportion of deaths in the 1918 flu pandemic.

Recent data has suggested that these two forms of pneumonia are not entirely unrelated. A study of 37,000 children in South Africa who received a pneumococcal vaccine found that they were on average one-third less likely to suffer viral pneumonia following infections with seven different respiratory viruses, as well as being protected from bacterial pneumonia afterward.

According to the World Health Organization, "Given the widespread presence of the virus...containment of the outbreak is not feasible. The current focus should be on mitigation measures." This means that preventing spread of the virus is not likely, and treating outbreaks will be important in minimizing the numbers of people who might become ill and potentially die.

Whether that is all there is or whether a person will become significantly ill is difficult to predict. Aside from people who are at risk, even perfectly healthy people can be infected.

At this point, how a community, a hospital, or an individual deals with the potential for infection will help decide how fast and how far it will spread.

In the face of a spreading disease, the importance of remaining calm is a point which cannot be emphasized enough. While something unknown can be a cause for concern, fear and eventually panic, the silver lining is that this is something which is not unfamiliar. It is a disease which has, although be it in slightly different forms, been documented in recent history. Hence, there is an understanding of what we can do.

Hence all it requires is calmness, a presence of mind and a mindset of 'preparedness'.

CHAPTER 4

Virus Structure

Influenza viruses belong to the Orthomyxoviridae family of viruses. The orthomyxoviruses have the potential to cause pandemics for their RNA is relatively unstable and keeps mutating all the time.

These viruses have the ability to adsorb on the mucoprotein receptors on the red blood cells (RBCs) causing haemaggluination. They also have an affinity for mucous lined organs, especially the respiratiry tract of hosts.

Single-stranded RNA viruses and RNA Sense

RNA viruses can be classified according to the sense or polarity of their RNA into negative-sense and positive-sense, or ambisense RNA viruses. Positive-sense viral RNA is identical to viral mRNA and thus can be immediately translated by the host ceil. Negative-sense viral RNA is complementary to mRNA and thus must be converted to positive-sense RNA by an RNA polymerase before translation.

As such, purified RNA of a positive-sense virus can directly cause infection though it may be less infectious than the whole virus particle. Purified RNA of a negative-sense virus is not infectious by itself as it needs to be transcribed into positive-sense RNA, however each virion can be transcribed to several positive-sense RNAs. Ambisense RNA viruses resemble negative-sense

RNA viruses, except they also translate genes from the positive strand.

These viruses are those which have only a single strand of RNA, which is of the antisense type. This determines whether the virus can directly use its RNA to manufacture proteins or whether it first needs to synthesisze a complementary strand which encodes the protein configurations

Types of Influenza Viruses

In virus classification, Influenza viruses are RNA viruses (belonging to Group V) that make up three of the five genera of the family Orthomyxoviridae:

- Influenzavirus A
- Influenzavirus B
- Influenzavirus C

These viruses are only distantly related to the human parainfluenza viruses, which are RNA viruses belonging to the paramyxovirus family that are a common cause of respiratory infections in children such as croup but can also cause a disease similar to influenza in adults.

Influenza Virus A

This genus has one species, Influenza A virus. Wild aquatic birds are the natural hosts for a large variety of Influenza A. Occasionally, viruses are transmitted to other species and may then cause devastating outbreaks in domestic poultry or give rise to human influenza pandemics. The type A viruses are the most virulent human pathogens among the three influenza types and cause the most severe disease. The influenza A virus can be subdivided into different serotypes based on the antibody response to these viruses. The serotypes that have been confirmed in humans, ordered by the number of known human pandemic deaths, are:

- **H1N1**, which caused **Spanish Flu** in 1918, and the **2009 Flu Pandemic**
- **H2N2**, which caused **Asian Flu** in 1957
- **H3N2**, which caused **Hong Kong Flu** in 1968

- **H5N1**, a current pandemic threat
- **H7N7**, which has unusual zoonotic potential
- **H1N2**, endemic in humans and pigs
- **H9N2**
- **H7N2**
- **H7N3**
- **H10N7**

Influenza Virus B

This genus has one species, Influenza B virus. Influenza B almost exclusively infects humans and is less common than Influenza A. The only other animals known to be susceptible to influenza B infection are the seal and the ferret.

This type of influenza mutates at a rate 2–3 times lower than type A and consequently is less genetically diverse, with only one Influenza B serotype. As a result of this lack of antigenic diversity, a degree of immunity to influenza B is usually acquired at an early age. However, influenza B mutates enough that lasting immunity is not possible. This reduced rate of antigenic change, combined with its limited host range (inhibiting cross species antigenic shift), ensures that pandemics of Influenza B do not occur.

Influenza Virus C

This genus has one species, Influenza C virus, which infects humans, dogs and pigs, sometimes causing both severe illness and local epidemics. However, influenza C is less common than the other types and usually only causes mild disease in children.

Properties, and Subtype Nomenclature

Influenzaviruses A, B and C are very similar in overall structure. The virus particle is 80–120 nanometers in diameter and usually roughly spherical, although filamentous forms can occur.

These filamentous forms are more common in influenza C, which can form cordlike structures up to 500 micrometres long on the surfaces of infected cells. However, despite these varied shapes, the viral particles of all influenza viruses are similar in composition.

These are made of a viral envelope containing two main types of glycoproteins, wrapped around a central core. The central core contains the viral RNA genome and other viral proteins that package and protect this RNA.

Unusually for a virus, its genome is not a single piece of nucleic acid; instead, it contains seven or eight pieces of segmented negative-sense RNA, each piece of RNA contains either one or two genes. For example, theInfluenza A genome contains 11 genes on eight pieces of RNA, encoding for 11 proteins: hemagglutinin (HA), neuraminidase (NA), nucleoprotein (NP), M1, M2, NS1, NS2(NEP), PA, PB1, PB1-F2 and PB2.

The H and N of the Virus

Hemagglutinin (HA) and neuraminidase (NA) are the two large glycoproteins on the outside of the viral particles. HA is a lectin that mediates binding of the virus to target cells and entry of the viral genome into the target cell, while NA is involved in the release of progeny virus from infected cells, by cleaving sugars that bind the mature viral particles. Thus, these proteins are targets for antiviral drugs. Furthermore, they are antigens to which antibodies can be raised.

Influenza A viruses are classified into subtypes based on antibody responses to HA and NA. These different types of HA and NA form the basis of the *H* and *N* distinctions in, for example, *H5N1*. There are 16 H and 9 N subtypes known, but only H1, 2 and 3, and N1 and 2 are commonly found in humans.

Each virus subtype has mutated into a variety of strains with differing pathogenic profiles; some pathogenic to one species but not others, some pathogenic to multiple species.

Variants and Subtypes

Variants are identified and named according to the isolate that they are like and thus are presumed to share lineage (example FujianFflu virus like); according to their typical host (example Human Flu virus); according to their subtype (example H3N2); and according to their deadliness (example LP, Low Pathogenic). So a flu from a virus similar to the isolate A/Fujian/411/2002(H3N2) is called Fujian flu, human flu, and H3N2 flu.

Variants are sometimes named according to the species (host) the strain is endemic in or adapted to. The main variants named using this convention are:

- Bird flu
- Human flu
- Swine flu
- Horse flu
- Dog flu
- Cat flu

Variants have also sometimes been named according to their deadliness in poultry, especially chickens:

- Low Pathogenic Avian Influenza (LPAI)
- Highly Pathogenic Avian Influenza (HPAI), also called: deadly flu or death flu

Most known strains are extinct strains. For example, the annual flu subtype H3N2 no longer contains the strain that caused the Hong Kong Flu.

Annual Flu

The annual flu (also called "seasonal flu" or "human flu") in the U.S. results in approximately 36,000 deaths and more than 200,000 hospitalizations each year. In addition to this human toll, influenza is annually responsible for a total cost of over $10 billion in the U.S.

The annually updated trivalent influenza vaccine consists of hemagglutinin (HA) surface glycoprotein components from influenza H3N2, H1N1, and Influenza B viruses.

The dominant strain in January 2006 is H3N2. Measured resistance to the standard antiviral drugs *amantadine* and *rimantadine* in H3N2 has increased from 1% in 1994 to 12% in 2003 to 91% in 2005.

Contemporary human H3N2 Influenza viruses are now endemic in pigs in southern China and can reassort with avian H5N1 viruses in this intermediate host.

Structure and Genetics

The Influenza A virus genome is contained on eight single (non-paired) RNA strands that code for eleven proteins (HA, NA, NP, M1, M2, NS1, NEP, PA, PB1, PB1-F2, PB2). The total genome size is 13,588 bases.

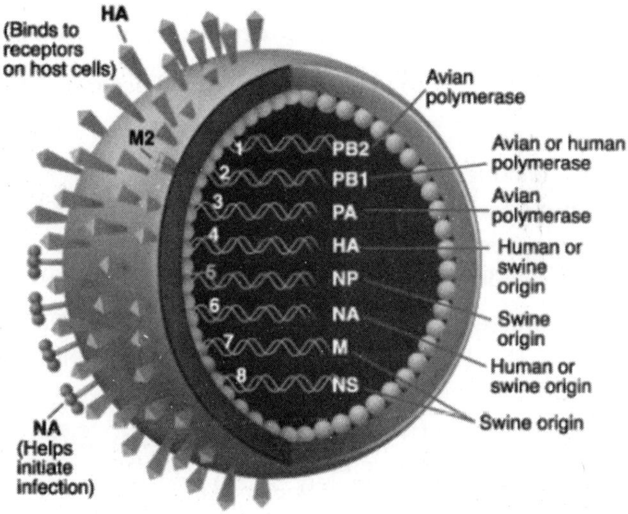

The segmented nature of the genome allows for the exchange of entire genes between different viral strains during cellular cohabitation.

The eight RNA segments are:

- HA encodes **hemagglutinin** (about 500 molecules of hemagglutinin are needed to make one virion) The extent of infection into host organism is determined by HA. Influenza viruses bud from the apical surface of polarized epithelial cells (e.g. bronchial epithelial cells) into lumen of lungs and are therefore usually pneumotropic. The reason is that HA is cleaved by tryptase clara which is restricted to lungs. However HAs of H5 and H7 pantropic avian viruses subtypes can be cleaved by furin and subtilisin-type enzymes, allowing the virus to grow in other organs than lungs.

- NA encodes **neuraminidase** (about 100 molecules of neuraminidase are needed to make one virion).
- NP encodes **nucleoprotein.**
- M encodes two **matrix proteins** (the M1 and the M2) by using different reading frames from the same RNA segment (about 3000 matrix protein molecules are needed to make one virion).
- NS encodes two distinct **non-structural proteins** (NS1 and NEP) by using different reading frames from the same RNA segment.
- PA encodes an **RNA polymerase.**
- PB1 encodes an **RNA polymerase** and PB-F2 protein induces apoptosis (or cell death) by using different reading frames from the same RNA segment.
- PB2 encodes an **RNA polymerase.**

The genome segments have common terminal sequences, and the ends of the RNA strands are partially complementary, allowing them to bond to each other by hydrogen bonds.

After transcription from negative-sense to positive-sense RNA the +RNA strands get the cellular 5' cap added by cap snatching, which involves the viral protein NS1 binding to the cellular pre-mRNAs.

The cap is then cleaved from the cellular pre-mRNA using a second viral protein, PB2. The short oligo cap is then added to the influenza +RNA strands, allowing its processing as messenger RNA by ribosomes. The +RNA strands also serve for synthesis of -RNA strands for new virions.

The RNA synthesis and its assembly with the nucleoprotein takes place in the cell nucleus, the synthesis of proteins takes place in the cytoplasm. The assembled virion cores leave the nucleus and migrate towards the cell membrane, with patches of viral transmembrane proteins (hemagglutinin, neuraminidase and M2 proteins) and an underlying layer of the M1 protein, and bud through these patches, releasing finished enveloped viruses into the extracellular fluid.

In Nonhumans

Wild fowl act as natural asymptomatic carriers of Influenza A viruses. Prior to the current H5N1 epizootic, strains of Influenza A virus had been demonstrated to be transmitted from wild fowl to only birds, pigs, horses, seals, whales and humans; and only between humans and pigs and between humans and domestic fowl; and not other pathways such as domestic fowl to horse.

Wild aquatic birds are the natural hosts for a large variety of Influenza A viruses. Occasionally viruses are transmitted from these birds to other species and may then cause devastating outbreaks in domestic poultry or give rise to human influenza pandemics.

H5N1 has been shown to be transmitted to tigers, leopards, and domestic cats that were fed uncooked domestic fowl (chickens) with the virus. H3N8 viruses from horses have crossed over and caused outbreaks in dogs. Laboratory mice have been infected successfully with a variety of avian flu genotypes.

Influenza A viruses spread in the air and in manure and survives longer in cold weather. It can also be transmitted by contaminated feed, water, equipment and clothing; however, there is no evidence that the virus can survive in well-cooked meat. Symptoms in animals vary, but virulent strains can cause death within a few days.

Highly pathogenic avian influenza virus is on every top ten list available for potential agricultural bioweapon agents.

Replication

Host cell invasion and replication by the influenza virus. The steps in this process are discussed in the text.

Viruses can only replicate in living cells. Influenza infection and replication is a multi-step process: firstly the virus has to bind to and enter the cell, then deliver its genome to a site where it can produce new copies of viral proteins and RNA, assemble these components into new viral particles and finally exit the host cell.

(a) Influenza viruses **bind** through hemagglutinin onto sialic acid sugars on the surfaces of epithelial cells; typically in the nose, throat and lungs of mammals and intestines of birds. After the hemagglutinin is cleaved by a protease, the cell imports the virus by **endocytosis** (i.e. engulfing it).

(b) Once inside the cell, the acidic conditions in the endosome cause two events to happen: first part of the hemagglutinin protein fuses the viral envelope with the vacuole's membrane, then the M2 ion channel allows protons to move through the viral envelope and acidify the core of the virus, which causes the core to dissemble and **release the viral RNA and core proteins**. The viral RNA (vRNA) molecules, accessory proteins and RNA-dependent RNA polymerase are then released into the cytoplasm. The M2 ion channel is blocked by amantadine drugs, preventing infection.

(c) These core proteins and vRNA form a complex that is transported into the cell nucleus, where the RNA-dependent RNA polymerase begins **transcribing** complementary positive-sense vRNA.

(d) The vRNA is either exported into the cytoplasm and **translated**, or remains in the nucleus.

(e) Newly synthesised viral proteins are either secreted through the Golgi apparatus onto the cell surface (in the case of neuraminidase and hemagglutinin) or transported back into the nucleus to bind vRNA and form **new viral genome particles**. Other viral proteins have multiple actions in the host cell, including degrading cellular mRNA and using the released nucleotides for vRNA synthesis and also inhibiting translation of host-cell mRNAs.

(f) Negative-sense vRNAs that form the genomes of future viruses, RNA-dependent RNA polymerase, and other viral proteins are **assembled** into a virion. Hemagglutinin and neuraminidase molecules cluster into a bulge in the cell membrane. The vRNA and viral core proteins leave the nucleus and enter this membrane protrusion.

(g) The mature virus **buds off** from the cell in a sphere of host phospholipid membrane, acquiring hemagglutinin and neuraminidase with this membrane coat. As before, the viruses adhere to the cell through hemagglutinin; the mature viruses detach once their neuraminidase has cleaved sialic acid residues from the host cell. Drugs that inhibit neuraminidase, such as oseltamivir, therefore prevent the release of new infectious viruses and halt viral replication. After the release of new influenza viruses, the host cell dies.

Since there is absence of RNA *proofreading* enzymes, the RNA-dependent RNA polymerase that copies the viral genome makes an error roughly every 10 thousand nucleotides, which is the approximate length of the influenza vRNA. Hence, the majority of newly manufactured influenza viruses are mutants, this causes **antigenic drift,** which is a slow change in the antigens on the viral surface over time.

The separation of the genome into eight separate segments of vRNA allows mixing or reassortment of vRNAs if more than one type of influenza virus infects a single cell. The resulting rapid change in viral genetics produces **antigenic shifts**, which are sudden changes from one antigen to another. These sudden large changes allow the virus to infect new host species and quickly overcome protective immunity.

Annexure I

GenBank Sequences of the H1N1 Virus

The following pandemic (H1N1) 2009 virus sequences were submitted to NCBI and are available in GenBank: *August 11, 2009, 7 submitted by Campus de la Universitat Autonoma de Barcelona, Spain; 96 by Public Health Agency of Canada:*

	PB2	PB1	PA	HA	NP	NA	MP	NS
Influenza A virus (A/Canada-AB/RV1531/2009(H1N1))	GQ465661	GQ465745	GQ465733	GQ465673	GQ465709	GQ465697	GQ465685	GQ465721
Influenza A virus (A/Canada-AB/RV1644/2009(H1N1))	GQ465667	GQ465751	GQ465739	GQ465679	GQ465715	GQ465702	GQ465691	GQ465727
Influenza A virus (A/Canada-NS/RV1551/2009(H1N1))	GQ465662	GQ465746	GQ465734	GQ465674	GQ465710	GQ465698	GQ465686	GQ465722
Influenza A virus (A/Canada-NS/RV1554/2009(H1N1))	GQ465663	GQ465747	GQ465735	GQ465675	GQ465711	GQ465699	GQ465687	GQ465723
Influenza A virus (A/Canada-NS/RV1565/2009(H1N1))	GQ465664	GQ465748	GQ465736	GQ465676	GQ465712	GQ465707	GQ465688	GQ465724
Influenza A virus (A/Canada-ON/RV1589/2009(H1N1))	GQ465666	GQ465750	GQ465738	GQ465678	GQ465714	GQ465701	GQ465690	GQ465726

(Contd.)

	PB2	PB1	PA	HA	NP	NA	MP	NS
Influenza A virus (A/Canada-PQ/RV1586/2009(H1N1))	GQ465665	GQ465749	GQ465737	GQ465677	GQ465713	GQ465700	GQ465689	GQ465725
Influenza A virus (A/Canada-PQ/RV1758/2009(H1N1))	GQ465668	GQ465752	GQ465740	GQ465680	GQ465716	GQ465703	GQ465692	GQ465728
Influenza A virus (A/Canada-SK/RV1788/2009(H1N1))	GQ465669	GQ465753	GQ465741	GQ465681	GQ465717	GQ465704	GQ465693	GQ465729
Influenza A virus (A/Canada-SK/RV1794/2009(H1N1))	GQ465670	GQ465754	GQ465742	GQ465682	GQ465718	GQ465705	GQ465694	GQ465730
Influenza A virus (A/Canada-SK/RV1797/2009(H1N1))	GQ465671	GQ465755	GQ465743	GQ465683	GQ465719	GQ465706	GQ465695	GQ465731
Influenza A virus (A/Canada-SK/RV2486/2009(H1N1))	GQ465660	GQ465744	GQ465732	GQ465672	GQ465708	GQ465696	GQ465684	GQ465720
Influenza A virus (A/Catalonia/63/2009(H1N1))	GQ464405	GQ464406	GQ464407	GQ464408	GQ464409		GQ464410	GQ464411

August 10, 2009, 112 submitted by WRAIR; 2 by Center for Disease Control and Prevention of Changsha, China:

	PB2	PB1	PA	HA	NP	NA	MP	NS
Influenza A virus (A/Bethesda/SP506/2009(H1N1))	CY044168	CY044169	CY044170	CY044171	CY044172	CY044173	CY044174	CY044175
Influenza A virus (A/Bogota/0466N/2009(H1N1))	CY044144	CY044145	CY044146	CY044147	CY044148	CY044149	CY044150	CY044151
Influenza A virus (A/Managua/0536N/2009(H1N1))	CY044152	CY044153	CY044154	CY044155	CY044156	CY044157	CY044158	CY044159
Influenza A virus (A/Mexico/48N/2009(H1N1))	CY044160	CY044161	CY044162	CY044163	CY044164	CY044165	CY044166	CY044167
Influenza A virus (A/San Antonio/PR921/2009(H1N1))	CY044192	CY044233	CY044234	CY044235	CY044236	CY044237	CY044238	CY044239
Influenza A virus (A/San Antonio/PR922/2009(H1N1))	CY044240	CY044241	CY044242	CY044243	CY044244	CY044245	CY044246	CY044247
Influenza A virus (A/San Antonio/PR923/2009(H1N1))	CY044248	CY044249	CY044250	CY044251	CY044252	CY044253	CY044254	CY044255

	PB2	PB1	PA	HA	NP	NA	MP	NS
Influenza A virus (A/Silver Spring/SP509/ 2009(H1N1))	CY044176	CY044177	CY044178	CY044179	CY044180	CY044181	CY044182	CY044183
Influenza A virus (A/Silver Spring/SP510/ 2009(H1N1))	CY044184	CY044185	CY044186	CY044187	CY044188	CY044189	CY044190	CY044191
Influenza A virus (A/Taiwan/T0724/ 2009(H1N1))	CY044193	CY044194	CY044195	CY044196	CY044197	CY044198	CY044199	CY044200
Influenza A virus (A/Taiwan/T1338/ 2009(H1N1))	CY044201	CY044202	CY044203	CY044204	CY044205	CY044206	CY044207	CY044208
Influenza A virus (A/Taiwan/T1339/ 2009(H1N1))	CY044209	CY044210	CY044211	CY044212	CY044213	CY044214	CY044215	CY044216
Influenza A virus (A/Taiwan/T1773/ 2009(H1N1))	CY044217	CY044218	CY044219	CY044220	CY044221	CY044222	CY044223	CY044224
Influenza A virus (A/Taiwan/T1821/ 2009(H1N1))	CY044225	CY044226	CY044227	CY044228	CY044229	CY044230	CY044231	CY044232
Influenza A virus (A/Changsha/78/ 2009(H1N1))						GQ463958		GQ463957

August 08, 2009, 4 submitted by Shin'ichi Shimada Saitama Institute of Public Health, Japan:

	PB2	PB1	PA	HA	NP	NA	MP	NS
Influenza A virus (A/Saitama/43/2009(H1N1))				AB514227		AB514228		
Influenza A virus (A/Saitama/55/2009(H1N1))				AB514226		AB514229		

August 07, 2009, 1 submitted by Center for Disease Control and Prevention of Changsha, China; 8 by Chinese National Influenza Center, China; 7 by CDC:

	PB2	PB1	PA	HA	NP	NA	MP	NS
Influenza A virus (A/Changsha/78/2009(H1N1))							GQ463196	
Influenza A virus (A/Hunan/SWL3/2009(H1N1))	GQ463197	GQ463198	GQ463199	GQ463200	GQ463201	GQ463202*	GQ463203	GQ463204
Influenza A virus (A/Mexico/4108/2009(H1N1))		GQ463207	GQ463206				GQ463205	
Influenza A virus (A/Mexico/4482/2009(H1N1))							GQ463208	
Influenza A virus (A/Mexico/4595/2009(H1N1))					GQ463209			
Influenza A virus (A/Mexico/4635/2009(H1N1))							GQ463210	
Influenza A virus (A/Mexico/4646/2009(H1N1))		GQ463211						

*This sequence has the H274Y mutation that might confer resistance to Oseltamivir.

CHAPTER 5

Treatment and Prevention

Why the Virus Spreads Quickly

Evidence from previous pandemics suggests that one person will infect about two others, and that flu spreads particularly rapidly in closed communities such as schools or residential homes.

People are most infectious soon after they develop symptoms, although they can spread the virus for up to five days after the start of symptoms (for children this is seven days).

The swine flu virus is spread in exactly the same way as the ordinary cold and flu viruses.

However, because few people, if any, have full resistance to the new strain, they are much more likely to become infected once they come into contact with the virus.

The virus is contained in the millions of tiny droplets that come out of the nose and mouth when someone coughs or sneezes.

These droplets typically spread about one metre (3ft). They hang suspended in the air for a while, but then land on surfaces, where the virus can survive for up to 24 hours.

Anyone who touches these surfaces can spread the virus on further by touching anything else.

Everyday items at home and in public places may have traces of the virus. These include food, door handles, the remote control, hand rails and computer keyboards.

People usually become infected by picking up the virus on their hands from contaminated objects and then placing their hands near their mouth or nose. It is also possible to breathe in the virus if it is suspended in airborne droplets.

While prophylaxis and further prevention seem like the next logical steps, it is extremely important that the disease be actually confirmed. This is necessary so that there is a distinction between those suffering from common cold and influenza.

This would also prevent the infected individuals from taking the medicines unnecessarily as they have numerous side effects. Such an act also ensures that the medication being available in limited quantity during an ongoing pandemic is not unnecessarily consumed.

Diagnosis

Thus the first step logically becomes the diagnosis of the disease in the laboratory. There are numerous methods for diagnosing influenza:

1. *Demonstration of the Virus Antigen*

A rapid diagnosis can be made by demonstrating the virus antigen on the surface of the nasopharyngeal cells by immunoflourescence.

2. *Isolation of the Virus*

Virus isolation can easily be done during the first 2-3 days of illness but less often during the later stages. Throat garglings are collected using a buffered salt solution, and treated with antibiotics to destroy any bacteria. These can then be isolated by inoculating them either in 11-13 day old eggs or in monkey kidney culture cells.

After incubation at 35 degrees for three days, the eggs are chilled and the fluids are harvested and tested for hemagglutination.

3. *Serology*

Complement fixation and hemagglutination inhibition tests can also be employed for the serological diagnosis of influenza. Complement fixation tests with RNP antigen of influenza viruses are useful as antibodies form only during infection.

Apart from these, detection of viral RNA by reverse transcriptase polymerase chain reaction is also very useful and extremely sensitive, but is of limited availability.

Treatment

In Swine

As swine influenza is rarely fatal to pigs, little treatment beyond rest and supportive care is required. Instead veterinary efforts are focused on preventing the spread of the virus throughout the farm, or to other farms.

Vaccination and animal management techniques are most important in these efforts. Antibiotics are also used to treat this disease, which although they have no effect against the influenza virus, do help prevent bacterial pneumonia and other secondary infections in influenza-weakened herds.

In Humans

Antiviral Drugs

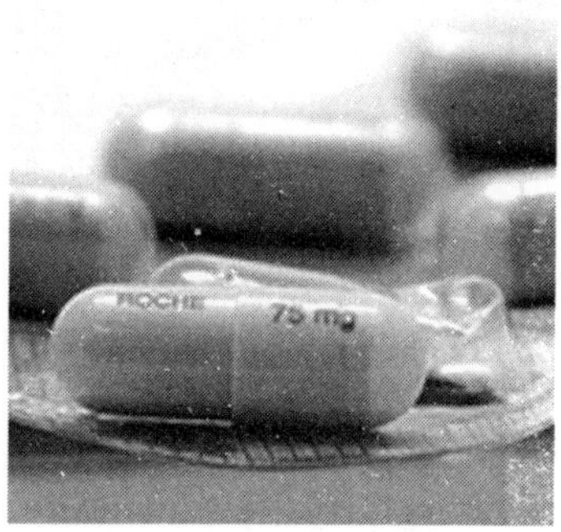

If a person becomes sick with swine flu, antiviral drugs can make the illness milder and make the patient feel better faster. They may also prevent serious flu complications.

For treatment, antiviral drugs work best if started soon after getting sick (within 2 days of symptoms). Beside antivirals, supportive care at home or in hospital, focuses on controlling fevers, relieving pain and maintaining fluid balance, as well as identifying and treating any secondary infections or other medical problems.

The U.S. Centers for Disease Control and Prevention recommends the use of *Tamiflu* (oseltamivir) or *Relenza* (zanamivir) for the treatment and/or prevention of infection with swine influenza viruses; however, the majority of people infected with the virus make a full recovery without requiring medical attention or antiviral drugs.

Oseltamivir is an oral medication, but zanamivir is inhaled through a device similar to an asthma inhaler and shouldn't be used by anyone with respiratory conditions, such as asthma and lung disease but is recommended for use by pregnant women.

The virus isolates in the 2009 outbreak have been found resistant to amantadine and rimantadine.

The U.S. CDC therefore recommends Tamiflu treatment primarily for people hospitalized with swine flu; people at risk of serious flu complications due to underlying medical conditions; patients at risk of serious flu complications because they are pregnant, under age 5, or over age 65; and to prevent infection of people at risk of serious flu complications who have been exposed to someone with swine flu.

In the U.S., on April 27, 2009, the Food and Drug Administration (FDA) issued Emergency Use Authorizations to make available Relenza and Tamiflu antiviral drugs to treat the swine influenza virus in cases for which they are currently unapproved. The agency issued these EUAs to allow treatment of patients younger than the current approval allows and to allow the widespread distribution of the drugs, including by non-licensed volunteers.

Antivirals are not a cure for swine flu, but will help to:

- reduce the length of time you are ill by around one day,
- relieve some of the symptoms, and
- reduce the potential for serious complications such as pneumonia.

It is especially important that high-risk groups get antivirals and start taking them as soon after symptoms start as possible.

Anti-viral Resistance Risk

Marie-Paule Kiely, WHO vaccine research director, said that it was almost certain that the new strain would undergo reassortment with resistant seasonal flu viruses and acquire resistance, but it was not yet known at what level resistance would appear.

If the virus develops oseltamivir resistance, the world's Tamiflu stockpiles will be worthless, and doctors would have to switch to the more expensive and harder to take, Relenza.

At least five recent instances of Tamiflu-resistant viruses were reported in July. There have also been reports of summer camps urging children to bring the antiviral drug Tamiflu and take it as a preventative measure, but that has concerned the CDC since widespread use could also lead to increased resistance.

Increased resistance to oseltamivir (Tamiflu), the leading influenza drug, has prompted federal health officials to change their advice about flu treatment, saying clinicians for now should consider using zanamivir (Relenza) or a combination of two drugs for patients suspected of having influenza A.

Currently, almost all seasonal flu strains are resistant to the drug and the genes for such resistance could be very easily transmitted to the new virus, the CDC warns.

Possible Side Effects

Both medications can cause side effects, including lightheadedness, nausea, vomiting, loss of appetite and trouble breathing and it is recommended that patients discuss possible side effects with their doctor before starting any antiviral medication.

The Food and Drug Administration (FDA) has required the maker of Tamiflu to include a warning that people with the flu, particularly children, may be at increased risk of self-injury and confusion after taking Tamiflu and that individuals with the flu who take Tamiflu be closely monitored for signs of unusual behavior.

Warnings of Online Purchasing

When buying these medications, some agencies warn against buying from online sources, with the WHO estimating that half the drugs sold by online pharmacies without a physical address are counterfeit.

Home Treatment Remedies

The Mayo Clinic and Medline list a number of ways to help ease symptoms, including adequate liquid intake and rest, soup to ease congestion, and over-the-counter drugs to relieve pain.

Aspirin, for instance, is very effective for treating fever in adults although in children and adolescents, aspirin is not usually given due to the risk of Reye's Syndrome (characterized by a degeneration of the brain, liver and kidneys).

It is important to remember though that while over-the-counter drugs relieve symptoms, they do not kill the virus. Most patients are expected to recover without medical attention, although those with pre-existing or underlying medical conditions are more prone to complications.

Prevention

Prevention of swine influenza has three components: prevention in swine, prevention of transmission to humans, and prevention of its spread among humans.

In Swine

Methods of preventing the spread of influenza among swine include facility management, herd management, and vaccination. Because much of the illness and death associated with swine flu involves secondary infection by other pathogens, control strategies that rely on vaccination may be insufficient.

Control of swine influenza by vaccination has become more difficult in recent decades, as the evolution of the virus has resulted in inconsistent responses to traditional vaccines. Standard commercial swine flu vaccines are effective in controlling the infection when the virus strains match enough to have significant cross-protection, and custom (autogenous) vaccines made from the specific viruses isolated are created and used in the more difficult cases.

Present vaccination strategies for SIV control and prevention in swine farms typically include the use of one of several bivalent SIV vaccines commercially available in the United States. Of the 97 recent H3N2 isolates examined, only 41 isolates had strong serologic cross-reactions with antiserum to three commercial SIV vaccines.

Since the protective ability of influenza vaccines depends primarily on the closeness of the match between the vaccine virus and the epidemic virus, the presence of non-reactive H3N2 SIV variants suggests that current commercial vaccines might not effectively protect pigs from infection with a majority of H3N2 viruses.

The United States Department of Agriculture researchers say that while pig vaccination keeps pigs from getting sick, it does not block infection or shedding of the virus.

Facility management includes using disinfectants and ambient temperature to control virus in the environment. The virus is unlikely to survive outside living cells for more than two weeks, except in cold (but above freezing) conditions and it is readily inactivated by disinfectants.

Herd management includes not adding pigs carrying influenza to herds that have not been exposed to the virus. The virus survives in healthy carrier pigs for up to 3 months and can be recovered from them between outbreaks. Carrier pigs are usually responsible for the introduction of SIV into previously uninfected herds and countries, so new animals should be quarantined. After an outbreak, as immunity in exposed pigs wanes, new outbreaks of the same strain can occur.

In Humans

Prevention of Pig-to-Human Transmission

Swine can be infected by both avian and human influenza strains of influenza, and therefore are hosts where the antigenic shifts can occur that create new influenza strains.

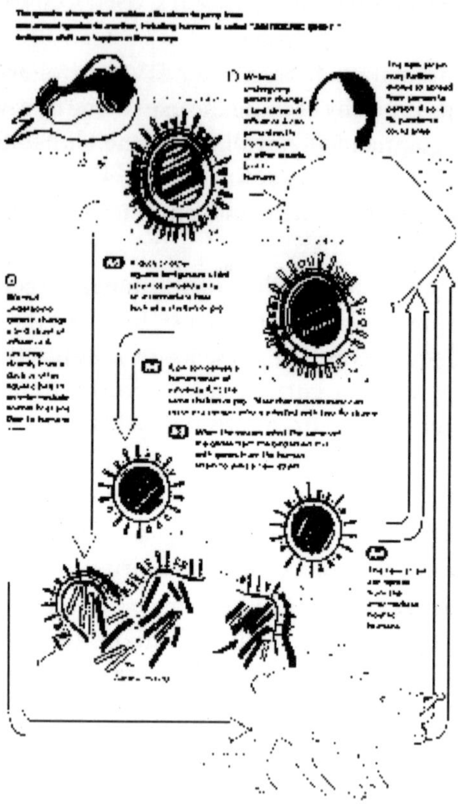

The transmission from swine to human is believed to occur mainly in swine farms where farmers are in close contact with live pigs. Although strains of swine influenza are usually not able to infect humans this may occasionally happen, so farmers and veterinarians are encouraged to use a face mask when dealing with infected animals. The use of vaccines on swine to prevent their infection is a major method of limiting swine to human transmission. Risk factors that may contribute to swine-to-human transmission include smoking and not wearing gloves when working with sick animals.

Prevention of Human-to-Human Transmission

Influenza spreads between humans through coughing or sneezing and people touching something with the virus on it and then touching their own nose or mouth.

Swine flu cannot be spread by pork products, since the virus is not transmitted through food.

The swine flu in humans is most contagious during the first five days of the illness although some people, most commonly children, can remain contagious for up to ten days. Diagnosis can be made by sending a specimen, collected during the first five days for analysis.

Personal Hygiene and Care

Recommendations to prevent spread of the virus among humans include using standard infection control against influenza. This includes:

- Frequent washing of hands with soap and water or with alcohol-based hand sanitizers, especially after being out in public.
- Mayo Clinic recommends a balanced diet with fresh fruits and vegetables, whole grains, and lean protein, sufficient sleep, regular exercise, and avoiding crowds.
- Chance of transmission is also reduced by disinfecting household surfaces, which can be done effectively with a diluted chlorine bleach solution.
- Use tissues to cover mouth and nose when coughing or sneezing
- Dispose off used tissues in a bin as soon as possible

Experts agree that hand washing can help prevent viral infections, including ordinary influenza and the swine flu virus. Influenza can spread in coughs or sneezes, but an increasing body of evidence shows small droplets containing the virus can linger on tabletops, telephones and other surfaces and be transferred via the fingers to the mouth, nose or eyes. Alcohol-based gel or foam hand sanitizers work well to destroy viruses and bacteria. Anyone with flu-like symptoms such as a sudden fever, cough or muscle aches should stay away from work or public transportation and should contact a doctor for advice.

Vaccination

Although the current trivalent influenza vaccine is unlikely to provide protection against the new 2009 H1N1 strain, vaccines against the new strain are being developed and could be ready as early as October 2009.

Avoiding Crowded Areas

Social distancing is another tactic. It means staying away from other people who might be infected and can include avoiding large gatherings, spreading out a little at work, or perhaps staying home and lying low if an infection is spreading in a community. Public health and other responsible authorities have action plans which may request or require social distancing actions depending on the severity of the outbreak.

Masks may be of benefit in "crowded settings" or for people who are in "close contact" with infected persons, defined as 1 meter or less by the World Health Organization and 6 feet or less by the U.S. Occupational Safety and Health Administration. In these cases the CDC recommended respirators classified as N95, but it is unknown whether they would prevent swine flu infection. According to mask manufacturer 3M, there are no "established exposure limits for biological agents" such as swine flu virus.

Pork Safe to Eat

The leading international health agencies stressed that the influenza viruses are not known to be transmissible to people through eating processed pork or other food products derived from pigs.

Airline Hygiene Precautions

Airlines around the world, particularly in the US have made no major changes as of the beginning of June, but continued standing practices that include looking for passengers with symptoms of flu, measles or other infections, and rely on in-flight air filters to ensure that aircraft are sanitized. The CDC has not recommended that airline crews wear face masks or disposable overcoats.

However, some airlines have modified hygiene procedures to minimize travel health risks on international flights. Asian carriers have stepped up cabin cleaning, installed state-of-the-art air filters and allowed in-flight staff to wear face masks, with some replacing used pillows, blankets, headset covers and headrest covers, while others have begun disinfecting the cabins of all aircraft. In China, some airline flight attendants are required to wear disposable facial masks, gloves and hats and even disposable overcoats during flights to select destinations.

Singapore has been thermal-screening everyone coming into the country, with Singapore Airlines giving passengers traveling to the United States health kits that include a thermometer, masks and antiseptic towels. Its cabin and flight crews are getting mandatory temperature checks before flights. The government recently quarantined a passenger who was later found to have the flu along with about 60 other people on the same flight who were sitting within three rows. A consultant for the microbiology division at National University Hospital in Singapore, said hygiene practices such as covering the nose and mouth when sneezing or coughing in confined areas may be the best way to limit infection and safety measures such as costly air filters may be of limited use for carriers.

Containment

On April 28, 2009, WHO's Dr. Keiji Fukuda said that it was too late to contain the swine flu. "Containment is not a feasible operation. Countries should now focus on mitigating the effect of the virus," he said.

He therefore did not recommend closing borders or restricting travel, stating that "with the virus being widespread... closing borders or restricting travel really has very little effects in stopping the movement of this virus."

However, on April 28, the U.S. CDC began recommending that people avoid non-essential travel to Mexico. Many other countries confirmed that inbound international passengers would be screened.

Typical airport health screening involves asking passengers which countries they have visited and checking whether they feel or appear particularly unwell. Thermographic equipment was put into use at a number of airports to screen passengers.

A number of countries also advised against travel to known affected regions, while experts suggested that if those infected stay at home or seek medical care, public meeting places are closed, and anti-flu medications are made widely available, then in simulations the sickness is reduced by nearly two-thirds.

Quarantines

Some countries began quarantining foreign visitors suspected of having or being in contact with others who may have been infected.

The Novel H1N1 Vaccine

WHO does not expect the swine flu vaccine to be widely available until the end of 2009, noting that current production yield was only about half as much as expected and would cause timeline delays.

Vaccine producers can normally produce about a billion doses of any single vaccine each year and as a result WHO anticipates a global shortfall.

There is also concern that countries which produce vaccines, 70 percent of which are in Europe, may delay sending swine flu vaccines to other countries as they may come under "tremendous pressure to protect their own citizens first."

Although WHO reports that a fully licensed vaccine might not be ready until the end of 2009, some experts feel that with little or no safety data about a swine flu vaccine, governments that are planning to roll out mass campaigns are taking a gamble, since any rare side effects won't show up until millions of people start getting the shots.

Nonetheless, in late July, some European countries were planning to accelerate the approval process for the vaccine, and countries like Britain, Greece, France and Sweden all say that they will start using the vaccine once it is given approval, which could happen within weeks. Some European officials feel that the benefit of saving lives is worth the gamble, and are letting companies skip testing large groups of people before the vaccine is approved. The U.S. however, is taking a more cautious approach.

U.S. and local health officials are monitoring the Southern Hemisphere, where the virus is already on an unstoppable course. Being winter there, it is feared that the virus might combine with the seasonal flu strain and develop drug resistance. The U.S. goal of pandemic plans is to make 600 million doses in six months, enough for two doses for each American, according to experts, with an estimated cost of $8 billion.

Although the seasonal flu vaccine provides little or no protection against H1N1 swine flu, health experts recommend immunization to help prevent people from being infected with both at once.

Two injections will be required three weeks apart for the swine flu and a third will be needed for seasonal flu to provide maximum immunity. Children younger than 9 years old will need four shots. The CDC plans to administer the vaccine through clinics set up by state health organizations, but some experts feel that health departments are under-funded and could get fatigued.

The groups recommended to receive the novel H1N1 influenza vaccine include:

- **Pregnant women** because they are at higher risk of complications and can potentially provide protection to infants who cannot be vaccinated;
- **Household contacts and caregivers for children younger than 6 months of age** because younger infants are at higher risk of influenza-related complications and cannot be vaccinated. Vaccination of those in close contact with infants less than 6 months old might help protect infants by "cocooning" them from the virus;
- **Healthcare and emergency medical services personnel** because infections among healthcare workers have been reported and this can be a potential source of infection for vulnerable patients. Also, increased absenteeism in this population could reduce healthcare system capacity;
- **All people from 6 months through 24 years of age**
  - **Children from 6 months through 18 years of age**

because we have seen many cases of novel H1N1 influenza in children and they are in close contact with each other in school and day care settings, which increases the likelihood of disease spread, and

- **Young adults 19 through 24 years of age** because we have seen many cases of novel H1N1 influenza in these healthy young adults and they often live, work, and study in close proximity, and they are a frequently mobile population; and,

- **Persons aged 25 through 64 years who have health conditions associated with higher risk of medical complications from influenza.**

It is not expected that there will be a shortage of novel H1N1 vaccine, but flu vaccine availability and demand can be unpredictable and there is some possibility that initially, the vaccine will be available in limited quantities. So, the ACIP also made recommendations regarding which people within the groups listed above should be prioritized if the vaccine is initially available in extremely limited quantities.

Once the demand for vaccine for the prioritized groups has been met at the local level, programs and providers should also begin vaccinating everyone from the ages of 25 through 64 years. Current studies indicate that the risk for infection among persons age 65 or older is less than the risk for younger age groups. However, once vaccine demand among younger age groups has been met, programs and providers should offer vaccination to people 65 or older.

Ayurveda

According to a news report, Ayurveda, the traditional 'science of life', has a remedy for diseases when every other stream of medicine fails. It has remedy for Swine Flu in the form of the miraculous herb, the basil leaves commonly known as *Tulsi*.

Tulsi has been known and worshipped in India for more than five millennia for its remarkable healing properties. Considered as an 'Elixir of Life', it has now been claimed to keep the deadly swine flu at bay and help fast recovery in afflicted persons. It had also proved useful in treating the Japanese encephalitis.

Apart from acting as a preventive medicine in case of swine flu, *Tulsi* can help the patient recover faster.

Even when a person has already contracted swine flu, *Tulsi* can help in speeding up the recovery process and also help in strengthening the immune system of the body, 'it is claims'.

Dr Bhupesh Patel, a lecturer at Gujarat Ayurveda University, Jamnagar is also of the view that Tulsi can play an important role in controlling swine flu.

"*Tulsi* can control swine flu and it should be taken in fresh form. Juice or paste of at least 20-25 medium sized leaves should be consumed twice a day on an empty stomach." This increases the resistance of the body and, thereby, reduces the chances of inviting swine flu," believes Patel.

Dr. Manikantan and Dr. Nisha Manikantan, senior ayurvedic doctors at Sri Sri Ayurveda centre have said, "Swine flu invades the body because of a breakdown in immunity. And Ayurveda offers simple & effective remedies to boost immunity & build resistance. Tea made from *Laxmi Taru* (botanical name: Simarouba) leaves, *Tulsi, Amla* and *Amrut* (Giloy) acts as an immunity enhancer. Alternatively & additionally, Ginger and Turmeric *(Haldi)* powder mixed with either lime juice or honey can also be taken twice a day."

"To counter air-borne swine flu viruses, *Sambarani dhoop* (loban stems) should be burnt in the house twice a day. *Sambarani* is a very potent atmospheric sterilser", the doctors added.

Scientific Prevention of Swine Flue has also been suggested using house hold products such as:

- Inhale Clove Oil *(Lavang)* For 1 Second
- Chew 1 Clove In a Day
- Eat Raw Garlic *(Lasun)*, Onion, Ginger *(Adrak)* (1 to 5gm)
- Drink Hot Milk With 2gm of Turmeric
- Consume Plenty of Vit C Fruits-Lemon/Amla
- Eat 8 to 6 leaves of *Tulsi* empty Stomach Twice a day
- Burn Camphor oil in your room, office: A little camphor oil all the time keeps different airbone diseases away

Annexure II

Pandemic Influenza Vaccine Manufacturing Process and Timeline

Pandemic (H1N1) 2009 briefing note

6 August 2009, GENEVA — It takes approximately five to six months for the first supplies of approved vaccine to become available once a new strain of influenza virus with pandemic potential is identified and isolated. These months are needed because the process of producing a new vaccine involves many sequential steps, and each of these steps requires a certain amount of time to complete. The vaccine development process from start (obtaining a virus sample) to end (availability of vaccine for use) is summarized below.

Activities at WHO Collaborating Centers

1. Identification of a New Virus: As part of a network set up for surveillance, laboratories around the world routinely collect samples of circulating influenza viruses and submit these to WHO Collaborating Centres for Reference and Research on Influenza for analysis. The first step towards the production of a pandemic vaccine starts when a Centre detects a novel influenza virus that differs significantly from circulating strains and reports this finding to WHO.

Vaccine virus is grown in eggs because the flu virus grows well in them, and eggs are readily available.

2. Preparation of the Vaccine Strain (called Vaccine virus): The virus must first be adapted for use in manufacturing vaccine. To make the vaccine virus less dangerous and better able to grow in hen's eggs (the production method used by most manufacturers), the virus is mixed with a standard laboratory virus strain and the two are allowed to grow together. After a while, a hybrid is formed which contains the inner components of the laboratory strain, and the outer components of the pandemic strain. It takes roughly three weeks to prepare the hybrid virus.

3. Verification of the Vaccine Strain: After its preparation, the hybrid virus needs to be tested to make sure that it truly produces the outer proteins of the pandemic strain, is safe and grows in eggs. Upon completion of this process, which takes roughly another three weeks, the vaccine strain is distributed to vaccine manufacturers.

4. Preparation of Reagents to test the Vaccine (with Reference Reagents): In parallel, WHO Collaborating Centres produce standardized substances (called reagents) that are given to all vaccine manufacturers to enable them to measure how much virus they are producing, and to ensure they are all packaging the correct dose of vaccine. This requires at least three months and often represents a bottleneck for manufacturers.

Activities at Vaccine Manufacturers

1. Optimization of Virus Growth Conditions: The vaccine manufacturer takes the hybrid vaccine virus that it has received from the WHO laboratories, and tests different growth conditions in eggs to find the best conditions. This process requires roughly three weeks.

2. Vaccine Bulk Manufacture: For most influenza vaccine production, this is performed in nine-to-twelve day old fertilized hen's eggs. The vaccine virus is injected into thousands of eggs, and the eggs are then incubated for two to three days during which time the virus multiplies. The egg white, which now contains many millions of vaccine viruses, is then harvested, and the virus is separated from the egg white. The partially pure virus is killed with chemicals. The outer proteins of the virus are then purified and the result is several hundred or thousand liters of purified virus protein that is referred to as antigen, the active ingredient in the vaccine.

Producing each batch, or lot, of antigen takes approximately two weeks, and a new batch can be started every few days. The size of the batch depends on how many eggs a manufacturer can obtain, inoculate and incubate. Another factor is the yield per egg. When one batch has been produced, the process is repeated as often as needed to generate the required amount of vaccine.

3. Quality Control: This can only begin once the reagents for testing the vaccine are supplied by WHO laboratories, as described above. Each batch is tested and the sterility of bulk antigen is verified. This process takes two weeks.

4. Vaccine Filling and Release: The batch of vaccine is diluted to give the desired concentration of antigen, and put into vials or syringes, and labeled. A number of these are then tested:

- For sterility
- To confirm the protein concentration and
- For safety by testing in animals.

This process takes two weeks.

5. Clinical Studies: In certain countries, each new influenza vaccine has to be tested in a few people to show that it performs as expected. This requires at least four weeks. In some countries this may not be required as many clinical trials were done with similar annual vaccine preparation, and the assumption is that the new pandemic vaccine will behave similarly.

Activities at Regulatory Agencies—Regulatory Approval

Before the vaccine can be sold or administered to people, regulatory approval is required. Each country has its own regulatory agency and rules. If the vaccine is made with the same processes as the seasonal influenza vaccine, and in the same manufacturing plant, this can be very rapid (one to two days). Regulatory agencies in some countries may require clinical testing before approving the vaccine, which adds to the time before the vaccine is available.

The full process, in a best-case scenario, can be completed in five to six months. Then the first final pandemic vaccine lot would be available for distribution and use.

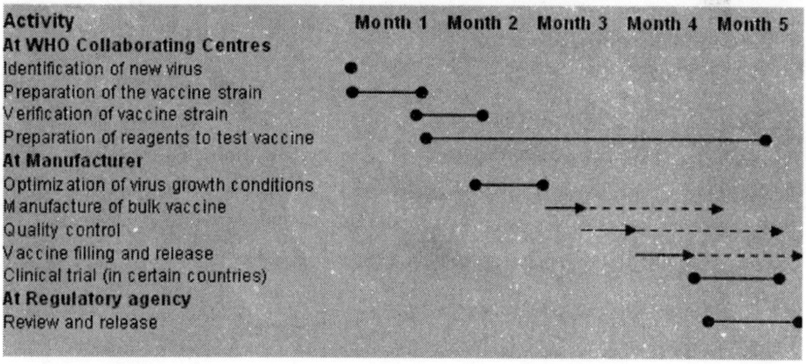

Key: The arrows with dotted lines preceded by non-broken arrows indicate the time period required for the first time an activity is done (non-broken arrow line) that is then repeated (dotted arrow line). The solid lines signify that the activity takes place within a finite period.

CHAPTER 6

Monitoring the Global Pandemic Situation

A Virus Emerges

Novel influenza A (H1N1) is a new flu virus of swine origin that first caused illness in Mexico and the United States in March and April, 2009. It is thought that this novel influenza A (H1N1) flu spreads in the same way that regular seasonal influenza viruses spread, mainly through the coughs and sneezes of people who are sick with the virus, but it may also be spread by touching infected objects and then touching your nose or mouth.

The first novel H1N1 patient in the United States was confirmed by laboratory testing at CDC on April 15, 2009. The second patient was confirmed on April 17, 2009. It was quickly determined that the virus was spreading from person-to-person. On April 22, CDC activated its Emergency Operations Center to better coordinate the public health response. On April 26, 2009, the United States Government declared a public health emergency and has been actively and aggressively implementing the nation's pandemic response plan

By June 19, 2009, all 50 states in the United States, the District of Columbia, Puerto Rico, and the U.S. Virgin Islands have reported novel H1N1 infection. While nationwide U.S. influenza surveillance systems indicate that overall influenza activity is decreasing in the country at this time, novel H1N1 outbreaks are ongoing in parts of the U.S., in some cases with intense activity.

Novel H1N1 Flu: A Pandemic Is Declared

On June 11, 2009, the World Health Organization (WHO) signaled that a global pandemic of Novel Influenza A (H1N1) was underway by raising the worldwide pandemic alert level to Phase 6. This action was a reflection of the spread of the new H1N1 virus, not the severity of illness caused by the virus.

At the time, more than 70 countries had reported cases of novel influenza A (H1N1) infection and there were ongoing community level outbreaks of novel H1N1 in multiple parts of the world.

Since the WHO declaration of a pandemic, the new H1N1 virus has continued to spread, with the number of countries reporting cases of novel H1N1 nearly doubling. The Southern Hemisphere's regular influenza season has begun and countries there are reporting that the new H1N1 virus is spreading and causing illness along with regular seasonal influenza viruses.

In the United States, significant novel H1N1 illness has continued into the summer, with localized and, in some cases, intense outbreaks occurring. The United States continues to report the largest number of novel H1N1 cases of any country worldwide. However, most people who have become ill have recovered without requiring medical treatment.

Given ongoing novel H1N1 activity to date, CDC anticipates that there will be more cases, more hospitalizations and more deaths associated with this pandemic in the United States over the summer and into the fall and winter. The novel H1N1 virus, in conjunction with regular seasonal influenza viruses, poses the potential to cause significant illness with associated hospitalizations and deaths during the U.S. influenza season.

CDC is continuing to watch the situation carefully, to support the public health response and to gather information about this virus and its characteristics. The Southern Hemisphere is just beginning its influenza season and the experience there may provide valuable clues about what may occur in the Northern Hemisphere this fall and winter.

Pandemic (H1N1) 2009 by country
Summary of official reports.‡‡

Country	**Cases Laboratory Confirmed‡‡**	**Deaths Confirmed (Suspected)**
ECDC total	215,090	1,735
Reports Total	**221,188**	**1,887**
United States	45,926	436
Argentina	5,710	338
Brazil	2,959	210
Mexico	17,581	149
Australia	27,663	98
Chile	12,030	97
Thailand	11,585	97
Canada	11,883	65
Peru	5,590	44
United Kingdom	12,261	41
Malaysia	2,253	38
Costa Rica	798	27
Paraguay	244	27
Uruguay	550	25
Ecuador	881	22
Colombia	275	17
New Zealand	2,984	14
India	2,401	36
Bolivia	1,022	12
El Salvador	626	12
Guatemala	558	10
Philippines	3,207	9
Spain	1,806	9
Singapore	1,217	9
Saudi Arabia	595	9
Honduras	263	6
Israel	2000	5
Dominican Republic	182	5
Hong Kong	5,991	4
Jamaica	64	4

(Contd.)

South Africa	1,300	3
Indonesia	771	3
Vietnam	1,211	2
Panama	600	2
Venezuela	476	2
Samoa	100	2
Taiwan	1,280	1
Netherlands	1021	1
France˜	880	1
Brunei	850	1
Ireland	475	1
Egypt	402	1
Qatar	350	1
Lebanon	210	1
Laos	156	1
Belgium	126	1
Hungary	125	1
Cayman Islands	88	1
Palestinian Territories	81	1
Iraq	67	1
Tonga	9	1
Mauritius	6	1
St. Kitts and Nevis	4	1
Ghana	2	1
Other	30,676	0

Surveillance Information

Influenza surveillance information answers the questions of *where, when, and what* influenza viruses are circulating. It can be used to determine if influenza activity is increasing or decreasing, but cannot be used to ascertain how many people have become ill with influenza.

Estimating deaths from influenza is also a complicated process. In 2005 influenza only appeared on the death certificates of 1,812 people (USA only). The average annual toll from flu is, however, estimated to be 36,000 (USA only). The CDC explains that "...influenza is infrequently listed on death certificates of people who die from flu-related complications." and furthermore that

"Only counting deaths where influenza was included on a death certificate would be a gross underestimation of influenza's true impact."

The last WHO update, issued on July 6, showed 94,512 confirmed cases in 122 countries, with 429 deaths. Many epidemiologists have pointed out that, in reality, millions of people have had swine flu, usually in a mild form, so the numbers of laboratory-confirmed cases were actually meaningless.

Partly as a result, on July 16, WHO announced that it will no longer issue the global tables showing the numbers of confirmed cases for all countries. Instead, national health authorities from all countries should inform WHO on a weekly basis of their qualitative assessment of the geographical spread, trend of cases, intensity of disease, impact on the health-care system, and deaths.

In the U.S. as of July 17, the number of confirmed infections was 40,617, with 263 deaths, according to the CDC. But the agency believes that more than one million people have been infected and were not tested for the virus or did not visit a doctor. Since the disease has now become so widespread, the CDC says it too will "probably" suspend counting cases within the next few weeks and focus instead on tracking clusters, severe cases, deaths and other unusual events.

Early Reports

The initial outbreak received a week of near-constant media attention. Epidemiologists cautioned that the number of cases reported in the early days of an outbreak can be very inaccurate and deceptive due to several causes, among them selection bias, media bias, and incorrect reporting by governments. Inaccuracies could also be caused by authorities in different countries looking at differing population groups. Furthermore, countries with poor health care systems and older laboratory facilities may take longer to identify or report cases.

The CDC in late May stated that counting confirmed cases had become "largely irrelevant," and switched instead to its traditional surveillance systems for monitoring flu-like symptoms by looking for patterns, clusters and changes in flu activity nationwide.

According to the CDC, surveillance methods, along with rapid isolation and treatment, only makes sense at the very earliest stage of an outbreak, and "becomes irrelevant" once the virus is spreading widely within the community, as it is in the United States.

In some instances, governments accused other countries of intentionally underreporting cases. Moscow, for instance, hinted that the Dominican Republic was under-reporting cases to "boost tourism." In early May, Cuba's Fidel Castro accused Mexico of hiding the scope of the epidemic until after President Obama visited the country in April.

Test Accuracy

In early June, WHO and the U.S. Food and Drug Administration (FDA) acknowledged that a new laboratory test used to identify the virus was about 90 per cent accurate, while rapid diagnostic tests have an accuracy of 50-70%. To be safe, some experts suggest, anyone who exhibits flu like symptoms (sore throat, cough, fever), should be presumed to have swine flu until there is concrete evidence to the contrary.

Raising the Alert Level

WHO had hesitated to raise its alert level and declare a phase 6 pandemic as the virus to date has caused generally mild symptoms, even though the pandemic level describes spread of the virus rather than its severity.

Having raised it to level 6 may cause many countries to adopt a variety of plans, such as shutting borders, banning events and curtailing travel. A move to phase 6 means that "emergency plans are instantly triggered around the globe."

In addition, at phase 6, many pharmaceutical companies may switch from making seasonal flu shots to pandemic-specific vaccine, potentially creating shortages of an immunization to counter the normal winter flu season.

Even though they have raised the alert level to the maximum, they are concerned that it should not create panic among the people.

WHO to Focus on Developing Countries

On June 12, the day after the pandemic was declared, WHO stated that its "primary concern is to strengthen and support health systems in countries with less resources." It emphasized that developing countries, where medical care systems are weak and supplies of antivirals insufficient will be the frontline of their battle against pandemic flu.

They also noted that even though the virus has so far caused mostly mild symptoms in rich countries, it could prove far more deadly to poor populations already weakened by malnutrition, chronic conditions like asthma and diabetes, or low immunity due to HIV/AIDS.

They were also working to make stocks of antivirals and antibiotics and an eventual pandemic vaccine more accessible and affordable to developing countries.

Northern Hemisphere

As of early July 2009, the flu has been reported in more than 100 countries, mostly in the Northern Hemisphere, with the United States reporting the most cases — more than 43,000, including at least 380 deaths, according to the World Health Organization.

As of May 30, 2009, seasonal flu is down, circulating at low levels; while the non-seasonal new H1N1 flu strain continues to spread and constitutes approximately 82% of all influenza viruses reported to CDC in the last week of May 2009.

Southern Hemisphere

In July 2009 WHO stated "The countries are seeing a mixed picture depending on the country. For example, in Chile, it was just reported that over 99% of their influenza viruses are the new pandemic H1N1 virus.

By contrast, in Australia, they see more of a mixed picture, where they are seeing both the pandemic H1N1 virus but they are also seeing a seasonal H3N2 virus that circulates there. In South Africa, right now the seasonal influenza viruses are much more predominant than the pandemic influenza viruses.

In the Southern Hemisphere, it is fair to say that there is a mixed picture. In another month or so, they will have a much clearer picture about how the pandemic virus is spreading in the Southern Hemisphere and whether it is beginning to crowd out the seasonal influenza viruses in many countries or in just some countries.

It is predicted that the virus is likely to continue spreading worldwide, especially in the Southern Hemisphere, where countries are in the winter months and the traditional flu season.

As of 6th August 2009, South America has had almost 30,000 laboratory-confirmed cases mostly in Chile, Argentina and Perú; and more than 700 deaths mostly in Argentina, Brazil and Chile.

On June 6, 2009, Australia's second largest city, Melbourne, was reported to be the swine flu capital of the world. On 9th July there were 1,876 cases in Victoria, including 11 deaths, mostly in Melbourne. However, according to Professor Robert Booy from the University of Sydney, the reason Victoria has the highest per capita rate of swine flu in the world "may simply be down to Australia's tough testing regime," and "is probably the best in the world at detecting this influenza virus." As a result, he feels that the U.S. and Mexico probably had more cases than have been reported.

In early June WHO and the U.S. Food and Drug Administration suggested that one of the testing methods used in Australia gives only a "presumptive positive" rather than a "definitive positive" result for H1N1 influenza and is only about 90 percent accurate. As a result, they stated that some Australians may have been given a false diagnosis.

In late June, swine flu was also detected in pigs at a farm near Buenos Aires, Argentina, but health officials there said the virus has not shown itself to be any deadlier to the animals than a normal flu. About a quarter of pigs at the farm were found to be infected, and veterinarians there are "very worried because humans are infecting the animals."

However, officials added that eating pork poses no danger to people. The discovery comes during winter in Argentina and the country is already experiencing a human swine flu outbreak with a death toll higher than any other country in South America. In

August, 2009, the first death in South Africa from Swine Flu was reported, a 22 year old man who died in late July.

An Interim WHO Guidance on Global Surveillance

Standardized and coordinated international information sharing is crucial for the management of the pandemic at global and national levels. National authorities need to know how the pandemic is evolving, not only in their own country, but also in neighbouring countries and continents. The continual flow and analysis of information provided by individual countries contributes to the development of a global picture that:

- Results in a better understanding of critical clinical, epidemiological and virological features of the (H1N1) 2009 pandemic
- Guides global prevention and control activities
- Allows healthcare providers and public health authorities to modify their own strategies for case management, community mitigation, and health resource allocation
- Reduces the impact of inaccurate and unconfirmed rumours

This guidance is going to remain valid until the end of 2009, for the time being. The CDC's new interim recommendations for healthcare providers include the following:

- Review local or state flu virus surveillance data weekly to determine which types and subtypes are circulating.
- Consider using rapid tests that can distinguish types A and B. Fiore said some rapid tests can do this, but others can't.
- Patients who test positive for type B can be given either oseltamivir or zanamivir if treatment is indicated.
- If a patient tests positive for type A, zanamivir should be considered if treatment is indicated. Oseltamivir should be used alone only if local surveillance data suggest that circulating viruses are likely to be A/H3N2 or B. A combination of oseltamivir and rimantadine is an acceptable alternative, and may be necessary for patients who can't take zanamivir, which is taken by inhalation and is not licensed for children younger than 7 years.

Amantadine can replace rimantadine if the latter is not available.

- If a patient tests negative on a rapid flu test, clinicians should still consider treatment, depending on local flu activity and clinical signs and symptoms. If treatment is indicated, zanamivir or a combination of oseltamivir and rimantadine should be considered.
- Where available, testing for viral subtypes can guide treatment. For patients with an H3N2 or B virus, either oseltamivir or zanamivir can be used; for an H1N1 infection, zanamivir or the combination of oseltamivir and rimantadine can be used.

What pushed the CDC to make the new recommendations, was the high level of resistance in the H1N1 viruses tested, plus the fact that most of the viruses tested so far this season have been H1N1.

Global Surveillance of Pandemic (H1N1) 2009 Virus Infections in Humans

The approach and methods for global surveillance vary at different stages of the pandemic. In countries with no or very few cases, the main aims of surveillance remain early detection of the introduction of the virus using laboratory confirmation of cases ad initial risk assessment.

In countries where the pandemic (H1N1) 2009 virus is established, the main aims of surveillance are continuous monitoring of the epidemiological, virological and clinical picture of the pandemic and its impact on the health-care infrastructure. Timely sharing of information is needed throughout the pandemic to enable ongoing risk assessment to take place.

A. Early Detection, Investigation and Risk Assessment

In countries with no apparent virus circulation the aims of surveillance are to document the first appearance of the pandemic (H1N1) 2009 virus and to collect sufficient information on initial cases for risk assessment. The requirements are to:

- Detect and confirm the spread of pandemic (H1N1) 2009 virus into areas, e.g. administrative units, not previously reporting confirmed cases
- Investigate changes in the characteristics of the pandemic such as any increase in the severity of the disease

Triggers/signals for the investigation of suspected cases or clusters of pandemic (H1N1) 2009 virus infection include:

- Cluster(s) of cases of unexplained initial infection or acute lower respiratory tract infection
- Severe, unexplained respiratory illness
- Changes in the epidemiology of mortality associated with the occurrence of lower respiratory tract illness, an increase in the number of deaths observed from respiratory illness or an increase in the occurrence of severe respiratory disease in previously healthy adults or adolescents and/ or among pregnant women
- Abnormally high levels of absenteeism in a school or workplace setting

The initial investigation should include laboratory confirmation of any suspected case of pandemic (H1N1) 2009 virus. Member States without laboratory capacity or with no access to laboratory capacity for confirmation, should contact their WHO regional office, so that an appropriate laboratory can be identified for the submission and testing of samples.

At any stage during the pandemic, unexplained clusters of respiratory disease or deaths, or any change in the epidemiological or clinical presentation of the disease seen to date, requires immediate investigation. The number of samples collected will vary depending on the needs of the investigation.

Reporting Requirements

Under the IHR (2005) Article 63, a State Party is required to notify WHO of the first occurrence of pandemic (H1N1) 2009 virus detected in their country.

Following this initial notification, the IHR (2005) subsequently requires the country to further communicate to WHO timely, accurate and sufficiently detailed public health information on the notified event.

WHO will continue to communicate directly with the IHR National Focal Point (NFP) to request specific information for risk assessment and risk management. Case definitions, laboratory results, source and type of risk, number of cases and deaths, conditions affecting the spread of the disease and the health measures employed should be included in this information.

The guidance below is intended to assist IHR National Focal Points and other national authorities responsible for gathering an providing such information to WHO.

At First Introduction of the Virus: Early Detection and Investigation

The first confirmed of pandemic (H1N1) 2009 virus infection detected in a country should be immediately reported by the IHR National Focal Point to the IHR Contact Point at the relevant WHO Regional Office as well as the WHO Country Representative where applicable.

WHO will follow established processes for internal communications about such notifications. Confirmed cases reported to WHO should be attributed to the country, territory or area in which they are identified.

At Any Stage during the Pandemic

IHR National Focal Points or national public health authorities should continue to notify WHO immediately on:

- Any changes in the epidemiological, virological or clinical presentation that are likely to be of significance for global risk assessment
- Any unusual or unexpected public health events, including clusters of severe unexplained acute respiratory illness or unexplained deaths due to respiratory disease.
- Mortality data: the number of deaths due to acute respiratory disease (by age group, if available).

B. After Detection of the Pandemic Virus: Description of the Epidemiology and Assessment of the Early Cases

Once the pandemic (H1N1) virus has been detected it is important to:

- Describe the epidemiological and virological features of cases to guide control and prevention activities as required
- Assess disease severity

Following the initial assessment of the early cases, the laboratory testing of a sample of suspected cases of pandemic (H1N1) 2009 virus is sufficient for ongoing virological surveillance. Laboratory sampling should then be directed towards:

- Confirming infection in new areas
- Testing severe cases
- Monitoring the co-circulation of pandemic (H1N1) 2009 virus and other respiratory viruses in countries with laboratory capacity for more detailed virological investigations.

For countries with limited laboratory capacity, or limited access to laboratory capacity, WHO recommends they aim to test a number of samples per week in order to verify that disease activity is still largely due to pandemic (H1N1) 2009 virus. For countries with laboratory capacity, detailed guidance is given below on virological monitoring during the pandemic.

Reporting Requirements

Initial Spread of the Virus:

Aggregated Case Counts and Descriptive Epidemiology of the Early Cases

After the first case(s) of pandemic (H1N1) 2009 virus infection have been notified and for as long as is feasible for the country, IHR National Focal Points or national public health authorities should report the following information to WHO on a weekly basis:

- The number of confirmed cases and deaths in confirmed cases

- The age distribution of confirmed cases and deaths (where available).

Countries should contact the relevant WHO regional office for reporting arrangements. A summary form has been developed to facilitate the reporting of this information to WHO. The WHO will use the information in accordance with Article 11 of the IHR (2005) as required by the circumstances of the pandemic.

In addition to the information asked above, all Member States are strongly encouraged to share with WHO any additional information relevant for ongoing global risk assessent. This includes, in particular, information on the clinical spectrum of the disease, the proportion of cases with severe illness, and risk groups for severe outcome.

Continuous Epidemiological and Virological Monitoring of Influenza Activity

Influenza-related activity should be monitored on a continual basis throughout the pandemic and should start as soon as possible, in all countries. At a minimum, countries should report on influenza activity.

The objectives of ongoing monitoring of influenza activity throughout the pandemic are to track:

- Global geographical spread
- Disease trend
- Intensity
- Impact of the pandemic on health-care services
- The number of deaths due to acute respiratory disease (by age group if available)
- Changes in viral antigenicity and antiviral sensitivity

Epidemiological Monitoring

Epidemiological monitoring will be carried out differently by Member States. Therefore, WHO monitoring activities will accommodate several types of data to allow countries at different stages of the pandemic to participate in this monitoring effort, regardless of their surveillance and laboratory capacities.

- **All Member States** are asked to provide a general

interpretation of information derived from a variety of information sources such as the geographical spread, the trend in the number of cases, the intensity of acute respiratory disease, and the impact on the health-care system.

ARI: Acute febrile respiratory illness (fever >38°C) with the spectrum of disease from influenza-like illness to pneumonia.

ILI: A person with sudden onset of fever of >38 °C and cough or sore throat in the absence of other diagnoses.

SARI: Meets ILI case definition AND shortness of breath or difficulty breathing AND requiring hospital admission.

Information sources for the qualitative assessment may include:

- sentinel sites for acute respiratory illness (ARI) influenza-like illness (ILI) and severe acute respiratory illness (SARI)
- absenteeism rates from schools or work places
- use of pharmaceuticals for symptomatic relief of respiratory disease
- outpatient or emergency department visits for acute respiratory illness—vital statistics indicating respiratory disease as cause of death
- formal and informal reports from district health authorities or health-care providers.

In Addition, Member States with established epidemiological surveillance systems will be asked to provide a set of quantitative numerical) data that can be derived from existing surveillance systems for respiratory disease, influenza or mortality.

Virological Monitoring

Global influenza virological monitoring is dependent upon the existing capacity of influenza virus surveillance and national capacity for virus detection and characterization. During Phase 6, the main objective of laboratory surveillance is to monitor the evolution of the virus for the purpose of:

- Detecting any genetic drift or re-assortment events that may affect virus pathogenicity
- Identifying drug resistance status
- Ensuring the specificity and sensitivity of current diagnostic assays
- Informing vaccine development.

Virological surveillance activities will vary according to existing laboratory capacities in terms of response, number of samples tested, number of samples selected for full characterization of the virus and many other factors. Accordingly, countries should respond in line with the following criteria:

Countries with a WHO designated National Influenza Centre (NIC), conducting regular seasonal surveillance are asked to provide WHO Collaborating Centres (WHOCC) with a representative number of isolates for further characterization and for use in vaccine updates or drug resistance monitoring.

Countries without a designated NIC but with ongoing existing influenza surveillance activities that have previously contributedisolates to WHOCCs for vaccine considerations, should continue to do so as category above.

Countries without a designated NIC and with no ongoing influenza surveillance activities but with capacity to diagnose the pandmic (H1N1) 2009 virus and/or other Influenza Asubtypes should follow their national guidelines for pandemic preparedness and the global surveillance guidelines in this document and send a representative number of specimens or isolates, depending on their laboratory capacity, to WHOCCs for further characterization.

Countries without a designated NIC, with no ongoing influenza surveillance activities and with no laboratory capacity to diagnose the pandemic (H1N1) 2009 influenza virus should collect representative samples from clinically compatible cases from newly affected areas and among severe cases. Each country should aim to collect clinical samples per week and send to neighboring countries or regional influenza laboratories with laboratory capacity for virus characterization. <Put in Four Boxes>

Countries should contact the relevant WHO Regional Office or WHO HQ for guidance on the collection, handling, and shipping of specimens.

Reporting Requirements

Unless other arrangements are in place between a Member State and the relevant WHO Regional Offices, the following reporting arrangements should be followed by national health authorities in collaboration with their National IH Focal Point:

- **National health authorities from all countries** should inform WHO on a weekly basis of their qualitative assessment of the geographical spread, trend of cases, intensity of disease, impact on the health-care system, and deaths.
- **National health authorities from countries with established influenza surveillance systems** should report on a weekly basis data on ILI and/or SARI
- **National influenza centres or reporting laboratories** are asked to report weekly via *FluNet* on the number of specimens collected and processed for influenza and the number of specimens tested that are positive for influenza by subtype.

In addition to notifications to the National IHR Focal Point, WHO has developed a surveillance system called *FluID* that can be used by countries to assist in reporting. The relevant WHO Regional Office should be consulted for further guidance on online access to *FluID*.

All national health authorities are encouraged to share with WHO any other information relevant to the ongoing risk assessment of this pandemic.

C. Analysis and Publication of Surveillance Data by the WHO

Data collected via WHO's global influenza A (H1N1) surveillance systems will be analysed and summary data will be published in graphs, maps and tables on WHO's web site and published in the *Weekly Epidemiological Record.*

WHO will use the information provided to inform global risk assessments, including mathematical modelling of the epidemic, to better understand the spread of the pandemic and the effectiveness of mitigation measures.

Scientists from countries providing data will be invited to participate in the development of, and be co-authors on, publications that draw on their country-specific data. Countries will always be consulted in the development of any articles in which their data has been used.

WHO will report and visualize the surveillance data provided. Reports will include alerts, situational summaries, tables, charts and maps of the evolving pandemic situation. The following graphics are examples of the outputs of WHO's global data collection.

There are numerous other collaborative efforts around the world to help monitor the 2009 H1N1 Pandemic:

Coordination Activities

- Collaboration in Response to the A (H1N1) Virus - Text En Espanol (Pan American Health Organization (PAHO) Representatives of several agencies of the United Nations system in Latin America and the Caribbean, together with PAHO Director Dr. Mirta Roses Periago, outlined the level of transparency and collaboration with which the Region is facing the spread of the new A(H1N1) influenza virus. Text in Spanish only.
- Influenza A (H1N1) En Español (World Health Organization) Get WHO guidance for national authorities, communities, health officials, and individuals. Provide daily situation updates and view outbreak maps.
- 2009 H1N1 Flu (U.S. Department of State) Contains press-briefing transcript on coordination efforts between the U.S., Mexico, and WHO.
- USAID Provides $5M in Emergency Support as Swine Flu Spreads (U.S. Agency for International Development).

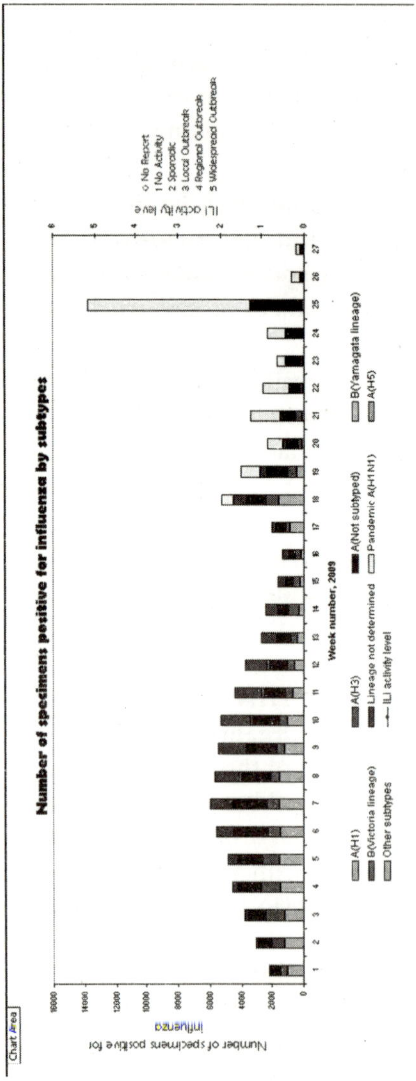
Chart Area
Number of specimens positive for influenza by subtypes
Number of specimens positive for influenza
Week number, 2009
ILI activity level
0 No Report
1 No Activity
2 Sporadic
3 Local Outbreak
4 Regional Outbreak
5 Widespread Outbreak
A(H1)
B(Victoria lineage)
Other subtypes
A(H3)
Lineage not determined
ILI activity level
A(Not subtyped)
Pandemic A(H1N1)
B(Yamagata lineage)
A(H5)

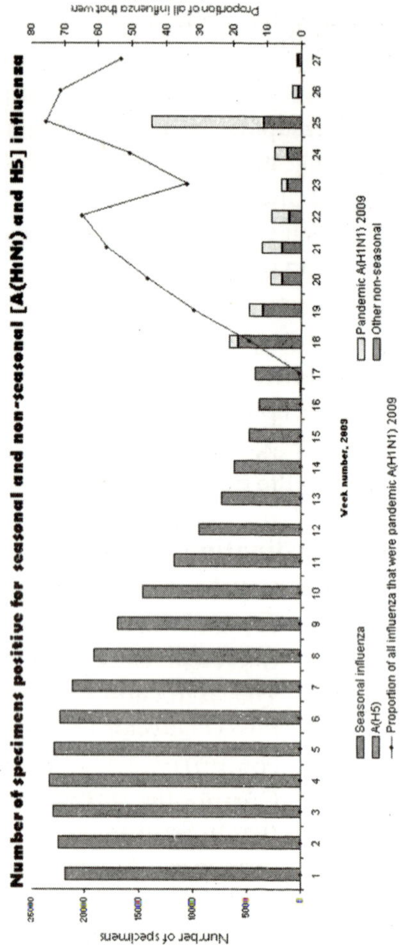
Number of specimens positive for seasonal and non-seasonal [A(H1N1) and H5] influenza
Number of specimens
Week number, 2009
Proportion of all influenza that were pandemic A(H1N1) 2009
Seasonal influenza
A(H5)
Proportion of all influenza that were pandemic A(H1N1) 2009
Pandemic A(H1N1) 2009
Other non-seasonal

- Influenza Technologies Available for Product Development: how HHS facilitates the worldwide development of new influenza technologies.

Global Monitoring

- Situation Updates and Maps - H1N1 Flu (World Health Organization) Global situation updates on the spread of H1N1.
- Timeline of Influenza A (H1N1) Cases (World Health Organization) This interactive world map shows the cumulative spread of new Influenza A (H1N1) cases as they were reported to WHO beginning 26 April 2009.

H5N1 (Avian Flu)

Coordination Activities

- U.S. to Provide Antiviral Medication to Latin America and the Caribbean for Novel H1N1 Influenza Control: U.S. will provide 420,000 treatment courses of Tamiflu (Oseltamavir) to the Pan-American Health Organization (PAHO) to fight the novel H1N1 influenza in Latin America and the Caribbean
- U.S. Government Support to Combat Avian and Pandemic Influenza (U.S. Department of State)
  This fact sheet outlines United States actions to support avian influenza preparedness efforts in more than 50 countries, in collaboration with the World Health Organization (WHO), Food and Agriculture Organization (FAO), the World Organization for Animal Health (OIE), and other international and in-country partners.
- Avian Influenza Action Group to Coordinate U.S. International Effort (U.S. Department of State)
  The Action Group will advance the international objectives defined by the National Strategy for Pandemic Influenza. The Group is also responsible for 83 specific actions to implement the U.S. international engagement strategy based on preparedness and communication, surveillance and detection, and response and containment.

- Avian Influenza: International Partnership to Meet a Global Threat (U.S. Department of State)—Read about ways that the U.S. is working with countries worldwide to combat avian flu.
- New Avian Influenza Flare-ups: Virus Remains a Global Threat (Food and Agriculture Organization of the United Nations)—Lists the new H5N1 outbreaks in poultry stocks in Bangladesh, Benin, China, Egypt, Germany, India, Indonesia, Iran, Israel, Myanmar, Poland, Russia, Ukraine, Turkey and Viet Nam.

Although there is no formal national surveillance system in the United States to determine what viruses are circulating in pigs, there is an informal surveillance network in the United States that is part of a world surveillance network.

Veterinary medical pathologist Tracey McNamara, set up a national disease surveillance system in zoos because the zoos do active disease surveillance and many of the exotic animals housed there have broad susceptibilities. Many species fall below the radar of any federal agencies (including dogs, cats, pet prairie dogs, zoo animals, and urban wildlife), even though they may be important in the early detection of human disease outbreaks.

Annexure III

Affected Countries/Continents

Africa

The **Egyptian** government ordered the mass slaughter of all pigs in Egypt on April 29, even though the current strain is a human-human transmittable, human influenza that has already previously hybridized with avian and swine flu. The World Organization for Animal Health called the swine killing "scientifically unjustified".

The first case of the novel H1N1 virus was discovered in Cairo, Egypt on the second of June, in a 12-year old girl coming from the USA with her mother. Only the girl was infected, and the officials caught the case before getting out of the airport. A second and third case were discovered on Sunday 7th of June, 2 students at the American University of Cairo.

On June 11, 2 more cases were discovered, bringing the total number of swine flu cases to 12 in Egypt.

The swine flu has been confirmed in 20 African countries: **Egypt, South Africa, Morocco, Algeria, Tunisia, Ethiopia, Ivory Coast, Seychelles, Cape Verde, Libya, Kenya, Uganda, Botswana, Zimbabwe, Tanzania, Mauritius, Somalia, Sudan, Namibia Zambia** and **Gabon**

Asia

Western and Central Asia

On April 27, **Azerbaijan** imposed a ban on import of animal husbandry products from America. AZAL took additional safety measures and a sanitary quarantine unit of the Health Ministry started to operate in Heydar Aliyev International Airport with all aircraft and passengers being checked.

On May 2 all checkpoints on borders with **Russia** passed to the medium security and disinfection barriers for both cars and pedestrians were installed at the Samur, Shirvanovka and Khan Oba checkpoints in Qusar and Khachmaz Raions. The veterinary services at checkpoints intensified their activities while hog farms in the northern regions passed to the closed farming regime.

Seventy-Seven cases have been confirmed in **Israel**. In response to the outbreak, the Israeli Deputy Minister of Health, Yaakov Litzman, suggested out of respect for the religious sensibilities of Jews and Muslims, the flu should be called "Mexican Flu." This was not done so as to not confuse the population into thinking that they could not acquire the virus if they did not eat pork. The Israeli government retracted this proposal following Mexican complaints.

The first confirmed cases of swine flu in **Kuwait** were reported on May 23, after about 18 people on U.S. military bases tested positive.

On May 30, three cases of swine flu were confirmed in **Lebanon**, the first in the country. "One Lebanese man who was in Spain and two Canadians who arrived in Lebanon a week ago are suffering from swine flu," the Health Minister said. They were put in quarantine and the blood samples that have been taken have proven to be positive.

The Lebanese Health Minister had previously asked citizens to stop the social habit of kissing. He also requested that affected schoolchildren be kept at home and that travel to countries in which cases have been confirmed be avoided. Beirut also banned the import of pork.

In **Saudi Arabia**, the first case of swine flu, which affected a Filipino nurse working at King Faisal Specialist Hospital and Research Center, was confirmed on June 1. The Health Ministry in cooperation with King Faisal Specialist Hospital and Research Centre has applied the national plan for the prevention of Swine

Flu in a manner that matches with the recommendations of WHO. Accordingly, the patient was isolated and provided with the required medical treatment. Arrangements are underway to examine those who were in contact with the patient to get sure that they are not infected.

Southern and South-Eastern Asia

Since 8 July, 2009 a total of 207 cases of Influenza A (H1N1) flu have been reported in **Brunei.** According to the Health Ministry, those who have been confirmed with Influenza A H1N1 will be given treatment as soon as possible and their close contacts will also be given treatment to prevent the infection. A 12-year-old girl who suffered from multiple chronic complications in Brunei became the first fatal case related to Influenza A (H1N1) in the country on July 2.

Cambodia's health authorities remain alert but confident that the country is prepared for a swine flu pandemic. In terms of ensuring that infected pigs do not spread the disease to Cambodia, the Cambodian Pig Raiser Association said it has told the government it should ban live pig imports. But Khlauk Chuon, the deputy director of Camcontrol at the Ministry of Commerce, said they would only ban live pig imports from a country that has been hit with swine flu.

All people entering **India** via the main airport hubs of Mumbai, New Delhi, Ahmedabad, Goa, Jaipur, Kochi, Chennai, Bangalore and Hyderabad are being screened. The primary focus is on passengers entering from the United States of America, The United Kingdom, Canada, Mexico, France, and New Zealand. As of 14th August 2009, over 1200 cases have been confirmed in India with 23 deaths.

The **Indonesian** Government halted the importation of pigs and initiated the examination of nine million pigs in Indonesia. Thermal scanners which can detect human body temperature have been installed at Indonesian ports of entry.

The **Lao** government bought ten thermal imaging machines to install at the country's major immigration border checkpoints. The Prime Minister said that masks should be made available and health officials would be assigned to work at border checkpoints. On 22nd July, Laos recorded its first death from Influenza A (H1N1).

In **Malaysia,** health screenings were carried out on passengers traveling to and from Mexico via sea, air and land beginning April 17. The Health Ministry's disease control division activated its operations room to monitor the swine flu situation and informed medical practitioners treating suspicious cases to inform the district health office immediately. Thermal scanners were installed at Kuala Lumpur International Airport. Screenings were imposed in Pengkalan Hulu, at the border with Thailand, in late April.

Quarantine rooms had been allocated in 28 hospitals, and the country has stockpiled more than 2 million doses of Tamilflu, as of May 2009. Schools were issued strict hygiene procedures on May 16 to contain any H1N1 outbreak among students and teachers.

On May 15, the Health Ministry confirmed Malaysia's first case of Influenza A (H1N1) infection of a male student who had arrived via air from Newark. Malaysia recorded its first local infection of influenza A (H1N1) involving the 19th case as that person had no history of having traveled to a country that had the flu. The first Influenza A (H1N1) related death was reported on 23 July, 2009. As of July 29, 2009 there have been 1,266 confirmed cases of Influenza A (H1N1) and 4 deaths reported in Malaysia.

In the **Maldives**, a ministerial committee has been established to supervise swine flu preventive measures to avoid an outbreak. All visitors arriving at the Malé International Airport on Hulhule Island and the country's three commercial seaports are being screened.

In **Myanmar**, the Chairman of Global Human Flu Prevention and Response Work Committee Deputy Minister for Health inspected preventive measures against the human flu at Yangon International Airport on May 1. Myanmar reported the first case of Influenza A/H1N1 in the country on June 27 with the 13-year-old girl who developed the symptoms after coming back home from Singapore a day earlier.

Pakistan has taken precautionary measures at the international airports to check passengers coming from swine flu affected countries. Doctors are checking the incoming passengers and allow entry only to those with no flu symptoms. The major hospitals in all the big cities are on high alert.

In the **Philippines,** thermal imaging equipment at airports was implemented to screen passengers coming from the US for flu symptoms. The Philippines may quarantine travelers arriving from Mexico with fevers.

Also, the importation of hogs from the U.S. and Mexico was manned, and the restriction of swine influenza vaccine use was retracted. On May 18, 2009, a Filipina girl who arrived from Houston, USA was the first confirmed case of H1N1 virus in the Philippines. As of June 15, 2009, there were 193 confirmed cases. By June 22, first known death was reported.

The first case of Influenza A (H1N1-2009) in **Singapore** was confirmed on May 27, 2009. It was announced on June 18, 2009 that Singapore appeared to have its first case of local infection of the Influenza A (H1N1) virus. As of July 9, 2009 the Singapore Ministry of Health no longer tracks the total number of Influenza A (H1N1) infections. The action was taken after the World Health Organisation told several countries that they were no longer required to submit regular reports on confirmed cases and deaths. As of July 7 there have been reported 1,217 confirmed cases of Influenza A (H1N1) in Singapore. As of July 25, there were 4 confirmed deaths related to Influenza A (H1N1) virus in Singapore.

On April 28, 2009, **Thailand's** Public Health Ministry issued a warning for Thais to avoid visiting the United States and Mexico which had been hit by the swine flu outbreak. The Thai Government installed thermal scanners in the Suvarnabhumi Airport and other key airports. Airport health officials began using thermal screening equipment to monitor passengers. Thailand raised its swine-flu preventive measures to "maximum", with all visitors entering the country subjected to thermal scanners and even dignitaries not exempt.

Vietnam's Ministry of Health released an emergency dispatch and urged agencies to take precautionary measures against swine flu. Thermal imaging devices were dispatched to airports and border gates to screen passengers. In response to WHO's warnings, Vietnam on April 30, 2009 raised its swine flu alert level to 4 which indicated a "threat of community level outbreaks" while local authorities have been executing precautionary measures. On May 1, 2009 an Vietnam's Ministry of Industry and Trade official said that Ministry was considering a ban on pork import "under certain situations" to prevent swine flu from entering Vietnam. As of May 31, 2009. The Government of Vietnam announced its First new case of A (H1N1) virus in the Country. A 23 years old Vietnamese student who recently returned from the United States has tested positive for swine flu.

Eastern Asia

On April 26, it was announced that that visitors returning from flu-affected areas to **China** who experienced flu-like symptoms within two weeks would be quarantined. May 2, the Chinese government suspended flights from Mexico to Shanghai. Meanwhile, the Civil Aviation Administration of China also assigned a charter to transport stranded Chinese visitors back home. The first suspected case found on mainland China was reported on May 10, 2009.

On April 29, the Food and Health Bureau of **Hong Kong** advised Hong Kong residents not to travel to Mexico unless absolutely necessary. The first case reported was a Mexican who flew in from Shanghai. The Bureau also escalated the alert level from "alert" to "serious", which activated health protection measures in all ports of entry of Hong Kong. As such, temperature-screening machines are used at all checkpoints to identify passengers with fever and respiratory symptoms. Any passenger who fails the temperature test and confirmed having a fever will be quarantined and sent to public hospital for further investigation.

Hong Kong also became one of the first jurisdictions to declare the swine flu as a notifiable disease, and much of the procedures against the spread of the swine flu were learned from the 2003 SARS outbreak, of which Hong Kong was the epicenter of the outbreak.

On May 1, one case became the first confirmed case of swine flu in Hong Kong and also the first in Asia. The Mexican patient arrived in Hong Kong on April 30. Metropark Hotel Wanchai, where the patient stayed, was quarantined. After the first swine flu case was confirmed by laboratory, Hong Kong's response level was raised from "serious" to "emergency".

In **Japan**, any live pigs being brought into the country were inspected to ensure they were not infected with the influenza. The Japanese Agriculture Minister Shigeru Ishiba appeared on television to reassure customers that it is safe to eat pork. The Japanese farm ministry said that it would not ask for restrictions on pork imports because the virus was unlikely to turn up in pork, and would be killed by cooking. On 8 May, the first three cases were confirmed. The infected patients had spent time in Canada and returned to Japan via Detroit. The first domestic infection was confirmed on 16 May in Kobe. As of 18 May, 130 cases had been confirmed.

South Korea warned against travel to Mexico City and three Mexican states. The government has also stepped up quarantine and safety checks on travelers arriving from the United States and Mexico, and pork imports from those countries. An emergency quarantine system is also in place, with simple tests conducted on people arriving with flu symptoms at airports.

On April 28, South Korea reported its first probable case of swine flu after positive preliminary tests on a nun who had recently returned from a trip to Mexico. Several sources have informed that one case has been confirmed by lab in South Korea, on April 30. On May 2, the first suspected woman turned out to be infected with the influenza A subtype H1N1. South Korea became the second infected nation in Asia.

On May 20, 2009, the first case of the influenza has been confirmed in **Taiwan.** The government had previously taken several steps to prevent the possible outbreak of Swine Flu, including a command center set up, travel alerts for infected nations, and more severe health check been conducted at international ports. Taiwan said visitors who came back from affected areas with fevers would be quarantined.

According to The Department of Health (DOH), Taiwan has a sufficient supply of surgical masks and vaccine to deal with the flu. The DOH also stated that they have 50 million to 60 million masks in stock and local manufacturers have the capability of producing 200,000 doses of the flu vaccine a month. In an effort to prevent the entry of the swine influenza, the Centers for Disease Control has announced on April 28 that every flight from the Americas, specifically Canada and the United States, that arrives in Taiwan from April 29 and onward will be subject to a strict on-board screening procedure.

On July 2, the first case of **oseltamivir-resistant virus** in Asia was announced in Japan, in a woman who had been taking Tamiflu prophylacticly.

On July 18, 2009, Hong Kong had its first swine flu **death.**

On July 3, a case of Tamiflu-resistant virus was discovered in a woman suffering from the flu. The woman had not previously taken Tamiflu, so concern has been expressed that she may have contracted an already resistant virus from someone else.

Europe

On April 27, the **Spanish** Ministry of Health and Social Policy announced that a man in Castilla-La Mancha who had recently returned from Mexico had contracted the disease. The man, aged 23, had returned from Mexico on April 22 and had been quarantined on the 25th. This was the first confirmed case in Europe.

On April 27, the **European Union** Health Commissioner advised Europeans not to travel to the United States or Mexico unless urgent. This followed the discovery of the first confirmed case in Spain.

On June 14, it was reported that the **United Kingdom** had its first confirmed swine flu related death. The individual was a Scottish woman.

As of August 8, seven countries in the EU (**Spain, the United Kingdom, France, Belgium, the Netherlands, Ireland and Hungary**) have confirmed deaths due to swine flu. Spain has four confirmed deaths; France, Belgium, Hungary, The Netherlands and Ireland all have one confirmed death, and the United Kingdom has 31 confirmed deaths (27 in England and 4 in Scotland) along with the British government suggesting 55000 new case of Swine Flu reported in the week up to the 16th of July 2009. The British government has also warned that deaths from swine flu this winter could be between 19,000 and 65,000 in the UK alone.

Hungary reported the first death in the country on 22 July. Ireland reported its first death on 7 August.

As of August 8, all European countries with the exception of the micro states San Marino and Vatican City have reported confirmed cases.

North America

A semi-logarithmic chart of laboratory-confirmed Influenza A (H1N1) influenza cases by date according to WHO reports. Mexico, USA, and Canada are shown as a breakdown of the total.

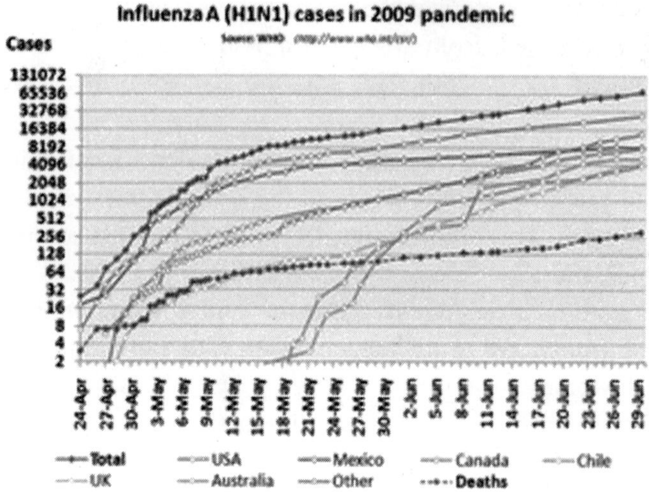

In **Canada,** as of May 26, there has been 16 deaths and a further 6457 confirmed cases of swine flu, most of which was contracted in-country, have been confirmed in the country; 68 in Nova Scotia, 114 in British Columbia, 86 in Alberta, 284 in Ontario, 106 in Quebec, 2 in New Brunswick, 6 in Manitoba, 3 in Prince Edward Island, 49 in Saskatchewan, and 1 in Yukon Territory. The country's first four cases, in Nova Scotian students who had traveled to Mexico, were confirmed on April 26. On April 30, the first case of swine flu affecting someone who had not travelled to Mexico was confirmed in Nova Scotia. On May 8, the first confirmed death from the H1N1 virus was reported in Alberta.

Dr. José Ángel Córdova Villalobos, **Mexico's** Secretariat of Health, stated that since March 2009, there have been over 1,995 suspected cases and 149 deaths, with 20 confirmed to be linked to a new swine influenza strain of Influenza A virus subtype H1N1.

Soldiers mobilized by the government have handed out six million surgical masks to citizens in and around Mexico City. On April 24, 2009, schools (from pre-school to university level) as well as libraries, museums, concerts and any public gathering place, were shut down by the government in Mexico City and the neighboring State of Mexico to prevent the disease from spreading further; the schools in Mexico City, the State of Mexico, and the state of San Luis Potosí remained closed until May 5. Marcelo Ebrard, Mexico City's mayor, has also asked all nightlife operators to shut down their places of business for ten days to prevent further infections.

On April 25, President Felipe Calderón declared an emergency which granted him the power to suspend public events and order quarantines. On April 26, the World Bank announced US$ 25 million in immediate aid loans to Mexico, an additional US$ 180 million for long-term assistance to address the outbreak, and advice on how other nations have responded to similar crises. On April 27, the Secretariat of Public Education announced that all schools in Mexico would remain closed at least until May 6. On April 28, the Mexico City government closed all restaurants and cinemas.

The National History and Anthroplogy Institute also closed all its archaeological sites and museums, including the most famous Mayan and Aztec ruins, until further notice.

In the **United States**, initial reports of atypical flu in two individuals in southern California led to the discovery of the novel swine flu virus by the CDC in mid-April. More than a hundred cases were confirmed in the next two weeks, spread through a dozen states. Outside of California and Texas, initial cases were all tied to recent travel to Mexico or close contact with those who had recently visited Mexico.

St. Francis Preparatory School, a private school in New York, was the center of a large cluster of cases after a Spring Break trip by several students, and became one of the first U.S. schools to be closed as a public health measure during the early outbreak. Most of the cases in California and Texas are not linked and may reflect localized outbreaks of this virus in those areas. The disease was not as virulent outside of Mexico as within Mexico, for reasons not fully understood. The US declared a state of Public Health Emergency but this was said to be standard procedure in cases as divergent as the recent inauguration and flooding.

On April 29, the US suffered its first confirmed death of swine flu, and on May 5 the first US citizen died from swine flu. As of June 6, there were 17 confirmed deaths from swine flu in the US. As of mid-May 2009 many states had abandoned testing for likely influenza cases unless serious illness and/or hospitalization were present. Since reported numbers represent only confirmed cases, they are a very great understatement of the total number of cases of infection, according to the CDC. The real number of swine flu cases in the United States could be upwards of 100,000; a top public health official estimated on Friday—far higher than the official count of 7,415 cases confirmed by laboratories. The United States now has more than 25000 confirmed cases and more than 140 deaths due to swine flu.

Caribbean

In **Aruba**, all passengers arriving by airplane or cruise ship were required to fill out a health questionnaire beginning on April 27, 2009. Hotels and resorts are required to report to authorities if any tourists are showing flu-like symptoms. The government of Aruba also ordered antiviral medication and other supplies from the Netherlands and the United States. No swine flu cases have been reported.

In **Barbados**, the first confirmed case of the H1N1 virus occurred on June 3, 2009. The second case was confirmed on June 6. The third case was confirmed on June 10. The fourth case was confirmed on June 17. Twenty-five outstanding samples have been sent to the Caribbean Epidemiology Center, the results of which would confirm if there is in-country transmission.

Cuba suspended flights to and from Mexico for 48 hours. The first case of swine flu in Cuba was confirmed in mid-May.

The first two cases in the **Dominican Republic** were confirmed on May 27. On June 5, a 17 year old pregnant girl infected with the AH1N1 virus died; 93 cases were confirmed to this date.

As of 7 July 2009, there have been 33 confirmed cases of swine flu in **Jamaica**. Health Minister Ruddy Spencer told Parliament that the country has been placed on high alert. There has been heightened surveillance at health care facilities and port entry's.

In **Trinidad and Tobago**, one female has been confirmed as having contracted the H1N1 influenza.

In the **Bahamas,** ten students and teachers who arrived from Mexico in the last week of April are in quarantine.

Central America

The first two cases of the flu pandemic in **Costa Rica**, both of whom had traveled to Mexico, were confirmed on April 28. As a result of a surge in new cases that occurred by early July, the Ministry of Health announced a new strategy to deal with this peak that resulted in increased deaths. Beginning July 11, 2009, testing for the virus will be conducted only on patients with risk factors and critical cases, including those with fever above 39 °C and patients with respiratory difficulties, as the main objective now is to reduce mortality rather than avoid contagion.

As of August 7 the Costa Rican Ministry of Health had 798 confirmed cases, 27 fatalities, 984 pending cases, and 4,630 already discarded. As of August 7 the official rate of infection is 17.9 per 100,000 people, up from 8 per 100,000 inhabitants before the first week of July when the contagion surge began. However, the mortality rate is still considered low, at 0,5 deaths per 100,000 inhabitants.

On July 21 the Ministry of Health, in agreement with the Catholic Church, and in order to prevent a massive contagion, prohibited the traditional pilgrimage to the Basílica de Nuestra Señora de los Ángeles (Our Lady of the Angels Basilica), patroness of catholic Costa Ricans. This pilgramage takes places every year on August 1 since 227 years ago, and this is the first time ever that is suspended.

On July 31 local authorities announced that the country was selected among the sample countries that will be part of the test of the vaccine developed by Swiss pharmaceutical Novartis. The local sample will include 784 Costa Ricans ages 3 to 64. Besides Costa Rica, this vaccine prototype will be tested also in Mexico and the United States. On August 11 was confirmed that Costa Rica's President, Óscar Arias Sánchez, was infected with the Influenza A (H1N1) virus, becoming the first head of state sick with the Influenza A (H1N1) virus. He will continue his regular work from home.

Guatemala is checking all travelers arriving from Mexico for signs of flu and stopping anyone with symptoms of the virus at border crossings. On May 5, in a meeting with Health Minister and the Vice President, it was announced that an 11-year-old girl was infected with the Influenza A H1N1 Virus. As of July 7 the Guatemala had 286 confirmed cases leading to two fatalities.

Honduras reported its first confirmed case of Influenza A (H1N1) flu on 27 May, 2009. By June 7 the country had reported 67 cases, most of the cases on the city of San Pedro Sula and the Atlantic Coastline. There are few cases on other cities and areas. All airports and commercial sites as well as public events are monitored. As of July 7 there were 123 confirmed cases and one fatality.

As on June 4, 179 confirmed cases had been reported by health authorities in **Panama**. Of these, 91 were male and 88 were female. Schools with positive cases are being disinfected. Thermal cameras had been deployed in Tocumen International Airport to identify sickness among arriving passengers.

As of July 7 **El Salvador** reported 319 confirmed cases, and **Nicaragua** 321. Panama and Nicaragua have not reported any fatalities.

Oceania

Australasia

The first confirmed case in Australia was reported on May 9. As of July 3, 2009, Australia has 7,290 confirmed cases. The first Australian death was on June 19 and the total death toll has risen to 20. The alert level has been lifted from "delay" to "contain", giving authorities in all states the option to close schools if students are at risk.

Australia has a stockpile of 8.7 million doses of Tamiflu and Relenza. At the beginning of the outbreak airlines were required to report passengers from the Americas with influenza symptoms, and nurses were deployed at international airports. Melbourne, the capital of the state of Victoria, is reporting the largest number of infections in the country, with Victoria having a higher per capita infection rate than either Mexico or the US.

On May 30, **New Zealand** had nine laboratory confirmed cases and 10 probable cases. All patients recovered. Over the month of June cases in New Zealand rose rapidly. On June 14 the Ministry of Health announced a 65% increase in cases in just 24 hours. On July 4, the Ministry of Health announced the first New Zealand deaths. There have been three confirmed deaths of patients who had tested positive for the flu; however two of them had known underlying medical conditions. The total number of confirmed cases has now reached 945.

Islands and Antarctica

No cases have been reported in **Antarctica**. Two cases were confirmed in the Pacific Islands. Both cases were confirmed on June 15, one in the **Solomon Islands** and another in **Samoa**. Five cases has been confirmed in **Fiji** as of June 24 and 1 case in **Vanuatu**.

South America

In **Argentina,** as of April 2009, passengers with influenza symptoms arriving from Mexico and United States were required fill out a form to be located should they experience any symptoms. In addition, the government has also stepped up safety checks, and thermal scanners are being used on airports to detect passengers with fever and other influenza symptoms. Flights from Mexico were also temporarily suspended as a precautionary measure. These measures however have proven to be largely ineffective.

As of June 22, Argentina had 1,213 confirmed cases of swine flu and 10 confirmed deaths, increasing to 52 confirmed deaths. The estimated number increased to as many as 100,000 affected people on July 2, as confirmed by the then newly appointed Minister of Health. As of July 14, the number of officially recognised cases skyrocketed, with 137 deaths, making the death toll in Argentina the second highest in the world, only behind the United States and surpassing that of Mexico.

As of April 2009, **Brazilian** airports have been monitoring travellers arriving from affected areas, under the direction of the National Sanitary Surveillance Agency (ANVISA). Aircrews were trained on signs and symptoms of swine influenza so that passengers displaying symptoms would receive guidance from ANVISA upon arrival. As of June 4, there were 28 confirmed cases of swine flu in Brazil.

The first case of Influenza A (H1N1) flu in **Chile** was confirmed on May 17. On May 29, the Chilean Health ministry confirmed the number of cases of A-H1N1 had risen to 224, the same day two more cases were confirmed. On June 3 Chile suffered its first confirmed death of swine flu, a 37-year-old man from Puerto Montt. Till date, and since the laboratory tests are no longer mandatory, the estimation of cases in Chile go up to 500.000 cases.

On May 3, 2009, the government confirmed the first case of Influenza A (H1N1) in **Colombia**, in a 42-year-old person from Zipaquirá, who recently travelled to Mexico. According to ministry, only one out of 18 tests sent to Atlanta was positive. The patient was isolated and put under medical treatment. On the same day, it was stated there were 108 suspect cases in the country. On April 27, the Government declared a "national disaster" state in order to face the emergency, which allowed health authorities to have a special budget to do so. The government purchased 400,000 oseltamivir (Tamiflu) doses, which would be distributed through the Social Protection ministry to the affected if there are confirmed cases.

Health officials are carrying out checks on people with flu symptoms entering the country from sea or air. On April 29, **Ecuador** closed its borders to Mexican citizens and foreigners of other nationalities arriving from Mexico for a period of 30 days. On May 15, Health officials confirmed the first case of AH1N1 flu in Ecuador. On May 20, the Health Department confirmed 7 more new cases of AH1N1, raising the total number of infected people to 8, the number has now risen to 41.

The first case of swine flu in **Peru** was confirmed on n May 14. On May 17, the second case was confirmed, an American-born man residing in Arequipa. He had returned from the US on May

12, not showing any symptoms until two days later. On May 18 a new case was confirmed, a scholar returning from a trip to Dominican Republic who had studied in the Altair school. Another case of a scholar from the same trip to Dominican Republic was also reported. The student had contact with a third victim and both studied in the same school.

The Governor of Callao ordered that all passengers from any infected country be checked before their arrival on Peruvian territory. Also, the Peruvian government must be warned of any case or symptom of fever. This step was in order to prevent any infections, since the main port and airport of Peru are located in Callao. Also, the government has prepared a special area at the Hospital "Daniel Alcides Carrión" to treat cases of this disease. Efforts have been made to examine slaughterhouses and they are screening incoming passengers from problem areas. All commercial flights from Mexico to Peru were suspended on April 29.

In **Venezuela**, controls have been raised at airports to prevent contagion from spreading. Travellers from the United States and Mexico with flu symptoms are being isolated until they are given the all clear. Pig farms in the country are being "closely inspected" and stockpiles of medicines built up. On May 28 the government confirmed the first case of the Influenza A/H1N1 flu in a Venezuelan citizen who had arrived in a flight from Panama. The following day, a second case was confirmed from another person who also arrived from the same flight.

Panic, Rush Leading to Reporting Bias

Epidemiologists caution that the number of cases reported in the early days of an outbreak can be very inaccurate and deceptive. This can be due to several causes, including selection bias, media bias, and incorrect reporting by governments.

One selection bias in epidemiology pertains to authorities in different jurisdictions looking at different sets of patient populations. For example, doctors in Mexico may be concentrating on patients in hospitals, rather than the larger vulnerable population, which may in part explain the higher mortality recorded in the country. Media bias in reporting swine flu cases and deaths may skew incidence maps based on these media reports.

Countries with poor health care systems and poor laboratory facilities may take longer to identify suspected cases, analyse those cases, and report them. Passive data collection methodologies (waiting for the patient to arrive at a health care facility) are considered inferior to active data collection techniques (performing random stratified sampling) due to various forms of selection bias and because laboratory facilities to perform swift genetic tests on patient samples are not widely available.

As of July 2009 there are no properly controlled epidemiological studies for the 2009 swine flu outbreak.

CHAPTER 7

Swine Flu in India

Current WHO Phase of *Pandemic Alert*

World Health Organization has officially designated the present outbreak as public health emergency of international concern and has raised the pandemic alert phase to level six implying widespread human transmission.

It has stated that containment may not be possible at this stage and is advocating mitigation measures. It has recommended against closing borders and restricting or banning air travel from affected countries.

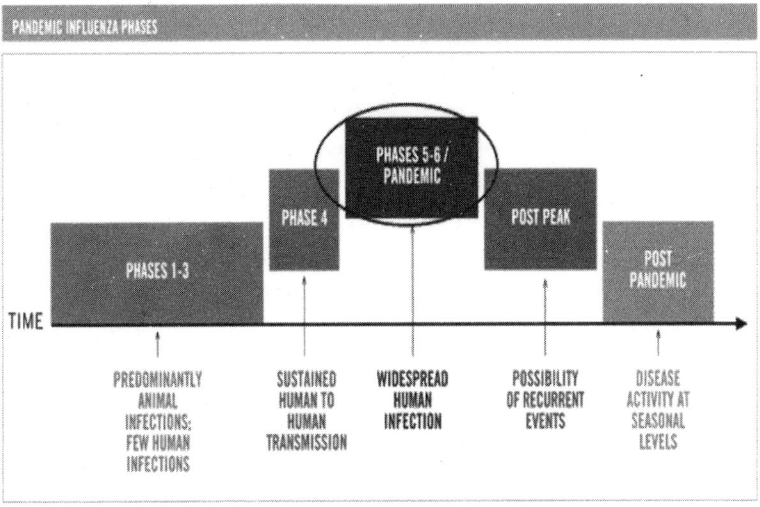

Situation in India

As of 29th June 2009, there was one imported case that came from U.S.A. With efficient human to human transmission established in case of the disease, and more than 48 countries involved at that stage, it was a matter of time before this pandemic strain would begin spreading. The behavior of this mutant virus among the Asian population is hard to predict. The virus has the potential to mutate further and become even more lethal.

The arrival of swine flu in India has caused panic in some areas. It has also led to concern about the ability of the country's health system to cope and even disrupted Bollywood.

Public concern about the spread of the Influenza A (H1N1) virus has mounted since the death last Monday of a 14-year-old girl in the western city of Pune, some 120 kilometres (75 miles) from the country's financial capital Mumbai. His was the first fatal H1N1 case in the country.

As of August 14th, twenty two other people who were confirmed to have the virus have since died, eleven of them in Pune, while more than 1,200 people have tested positive, the health ministry said.

But there were appeals for calm as green surgical face masks become a more common sight, including in the crowd at the World Badminton Championships in Hyderabad where a Malaysia coach has been tested for the virus.

India's Health Minister Ghulam Nabi Azad has stressed that swine flu should be put in the context of other health risks in the country. According to him, there were many fatal and costlier diseases circulating in the country.

With most confirmed cases so far among people who have returned from overseas, tens of thousands of travellers arriving at India's 22 international airports from affected countries have been screened.

A 24-hour helpline and website have been set up, public hospitals have been given responsibility for testing, isolation and management of suspected cases and 100,000 doses of the anti-viral drug Tamiflu have been sent to affected cities.

With the monsoon season in full swing, and the possibility of the administration being unprepared to tackle problems such as water-logging etc, the fears of acquiring other typical diseases is also paramount.

More than anything though, many have blamed the media for fuelling the fears about the lethality of the H1N1 flu among the masses even more. India's fiercely competitive cable news channels have devoted hours of airtime to the virus daily, frequently featuring reporters wearing masks stood in front of long lines of people waiting outside hospitals.

There has been a general appeal from authorities to the people to remain calm and not panic. They have sought to use the print and electronic media as well as the internet to educate the general public about preventive measures they can take. They have also tried to tell the people that the disease is not lethal, and fatality has been attributed to a previously exiting medical condition.

In a sign of the disruption, however, top Bollywood film director Karan Johar cancelled a planned shoot for his next movie in Pune, where a cluster of Influenza A (H1N1) cases has seen schools, cinemas and shopping malls shut.

There have also been reports of cancellations in the leisure and tourism sector.

As many public hospitals have overwhelmed with worried people, the parents of the country's first victim accused doctors of criminal negligence and demanded 50 million rupees (one million dollars) in compensation for alleged delays and mistakes in her treatment.

Meanwhile, at least three states, including Maharashtra, of which Mumbai is the capital, and Delhi, have invoked emergency powers to force anyone showing symptoms of swine flu to be tested for the virus.

The World Health Organization said on August 11th that nearly 1,150 people had died since swine flu first emerged in Mexico and the United States in April, while there were more than 177,000 confirmed infections.

That compares with 250,000 to 500,000 deaths and between three million to five million cases of severe illness from seasonal flu each year.

Dr Saradha Suresh, a pediatrician and member of the Indian Clinical Epidemiology Network, said in that context, Indians' fears were exaggerated.

"Mortality is only one to two percent, maybe increasing later... If you're looking at tuberculosis and malaria, we have more deaths than swine flu," she told AFP from the southern city of Chennai.

Swine flu, however, has been hogging all attention because it is unknown. It is expected that some 8000-9000 people are likely to catch the virus in the coming days and weeks through secondary contact with carriers.

When people actually need to worry is if they have some illnesses like asthma.

Meanwhile schools, malls and cinema halls in some cities in western India have shut and Bollywood shoots cancelled as the toll from the H1N1 pandemic rose to eight.

A Shutdown

More than 850 have so far tested positive for the virus, Health Minister Ghulam Nabi Azad said, with about 340 still undergoing treatment and the rest discharged from hospitals.

India was importing more supplies of flu drug Tamiflu and testing kits, asking private hospitals to help state-run hospitals cope with a surge in people rushing to get tested.

The flu drug is still supplied only by the state and will not be made available in pharmacies, Azad said. Three Indian drug firms were working on a vaccine, although it could take 5-7 months to make one available, he said.

In western Maharashtra state, which has six of the eight fatalities so far, schools, malls and cinema halls in Pune city have shut and companies are restricting travel to and from the industrial hub, about 180 km from Mumbai.

A team from the National Institute of Communicable Diseases was in the state to check the formation of clusters, the Indian Express paper said, citing a state health official.

H1N1 swine flu is unstoppable, according to the World Health Organisation, which has given up on trying to keep a precise count of cases.

Experts consider the pandemic to be moderate at this point, meaning it can kill people and put many in hospital, sometimes with severe illness. But most people get a mild illness and get better with little or no treatment.

In Mumbai, commuters on crowded local trains wore face masks or handkerchiefs, and several pharmacies were selling swine flu masks and hand sanitisers at several times the regular price.

Several schools have closed for a week; although Azad said simply closing schools would not help contain the virus if children chose instead to go to the mall or to parties.

Investors are worried and Mumbai's benchmark Sensex has caught a bit of a fever. It has lost 6% since August 3 falling 915 points to 15,009 yesterday, though today's morning trading showed some signs of recovery.

Panic Attacks

The creeping death toll has caused a panicky populace to flock to government-run hospitals to get themselves screened for the virus. The collected samples are sent to designated state-owned labs for testing. Such is the rush that the federal government has recently permitted private hospitals and labs to pitch in.

Swine flu is already a global pandemic, with more than 160,000 cases and 1,154 deaths recorded worldwide, according to the World Health Organization. In fact, swine flu hit India later than many countries.

Since it is a new virus, no one in the world had immunity to it when it came on the scene earlier this year, so it is spreading quickly. Fortunately it has proved a relatively mild flu for most people.

Meanwhile, the government, in a bid to pacify the anxious population has also announced that Swine Flu would be covered under all major mediclaim policies.

Rush for Vaccine

Drugmakers around the world are rushing to produce the swine flu vaccine by this fall.

While three Indian firms have already begun working to develop the swine flu vaccine, the minister has stated that the country will import the vaccine until the local version becomes available. Suresh Jadhav, executive director of Serum Institute of India, one of the three firms racing to make the vaccine, said that he expects to send a batch for testing by September and phase 1 clinical trials should start by January. In a best-case scenario, the earliest Serum's vaccine would be available in the market is April, said Jadhav.

Serum has no assured orders for the vaccine from the government so far, but Cyrus Poonawalla, who owns the firm, which is located in Pune, has decided to set up a manufacturing facility in anticipation of future demand-and hopefully windfall profits.

CHAPTER 8

Government of India Action Plan

Phase-wise Approach

India had been following a phase-wise approach advocated by World Health Organization for averting avian influenza and for containment of a novel virus that could emerge and eventually get adapted for efficient human-to-human transmission.

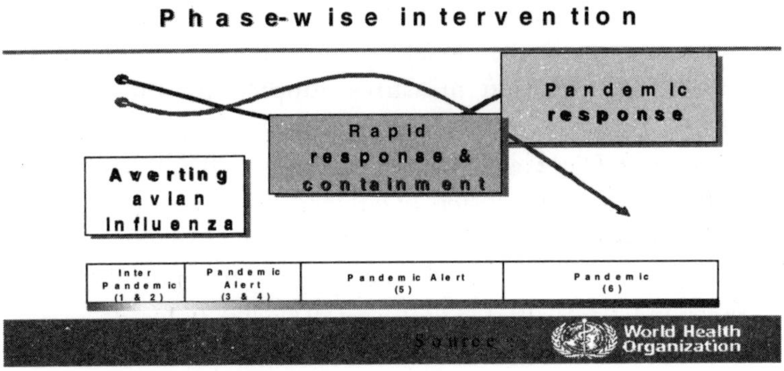

For the present pandemic with re-assorted influenza A H1N1, as of now, WHO is not advocating a containment strategy. It is also not known how this virus or a further mutated strain would behave in Indian population.

Strategy

The phase 5/6 requires substantial action from sectors other than health that would be coordinated by NDMA. These actions will culminate in weaving the entire set of actions into the national disaster management framework for phase-6.

The strategic approach for health sector revolves around five broad areas of—

(i) Surveillance and early detection
(ii) Pharmaceutical intervention and
(iii) Non-Pharmaceutical intervention
(iv) Clinical management
(v) Risk communication

(i) Surveillance

Existing surveillance mechanisms at community level, ports and airports and border crossings would be strengthened to detect early clusters of influenza-like illness or severe acute respiratory illness. The laboratory (virological) surveillance need to detect the circulating strains and should have the capability to detect any new strain that enters the country or gets established within the country.

India would network with WHO and the global influenza networks to monitor the global situation and to understand the containment/mitigation measures adopted by the affected countries.

Integrated Disease Surveillance Project (IDSP) would be strengthened to report clusters of influenza like illness (ILI) in real time. The medical practitioners, both in Government and non governmental sector would also be appealed to report ILI.

When India gets affected with a small cluster and transmission is not efficient, cluster containment strategy could be enforced provided it is supported by the requisite legal, administrative, technical and resource support. The defined population in a geographic area would be subjected to active house-to-house surveillance, contact tracing and chemoprophylaxis.

If wide spread infection is inevitable, then the health care institutions would be reporting the morbidity and mortality.

(ii) Pharmaceutical Intervention

As of now, India has a stock of 10 million capsules of oseltamivir. Some stocks are also committed by pharmaceutical companies for exclusive use by the Government. This drug is only available through the public health system and its retail sale is banned as indiscriminate use may lead to development of resistance. If there is widespread infection, MOHFW would review this decision.

(a) Oseltamivir

Treatment

- At the individual level, Oseltamivir would be used to treat cases.
- Initially oseltamivir is recommended to be given to all suspect cases and to provide chemoprophylaxis to immediate family and social contacts. Once the infection gets widespread but with less severity, then oseltamivir need to be provided only to those developing lower respiratory tract infection

Chemoprophylaxis

- Chemoprophylaxis for health care workers at high risk
  - The treating physicians and other paramedical personnel at the isolation facility would be put on chemoprophylaxis.
- Chemoprophylaxis for contacts
  - Chemoprophylaxis is advised for those contacts with high risk (with under lying systemic diseases; extremes of age [< 5 years and > 65 Years].
  - In phase -5, if the clusters are reported for the first time, and given that those exposed are known and can be traced easily, then family, social and community contacts should be given chemoprophylaxis.
- Mass Chemoprophylaxis:
- The strategy of containment by geographic approach by giving oseltamivir to every individual in a prescribed geographic limit of 5 km from the epicenter (The village /

city where the cluster is reported) would be applied :

- If the virus is lethal and causing severe morbidity and high mortality and
- Though effecting humans, is not efficiently transmitting in our population and
- If the cluster is limited by natural geographic boundaries

A direct inference to this effect can be drawn from the time line with in which number of secondary cases emerges from the primary case. One such indicator is the reproductive number; if one person infects two persons in 3 days (15 cases in 10 days) containment may be difficult but yet possible. If the spread is more than this, containment is less likely.

Widely dispersed multiple clusters would indicate that the clusters cannot be contained through the geographic approach. District Collector would be informed of this by the Central / State RRT. This strategic decision would be taken by the RRT in consultation with State Health Department/ MOHFW, Government of India.

(b) Influenza H1N1 Vaccine

The currently available information suggests that seasonal influenza vaccine is found not effective against the re-assorted virus. It takes about six months to manufacture a vaccine against a novel virus. Hence, a vaccine may not be available during the first wave of the pandemic. If the candidate vaccine strains are made available by WHO or synthesized in our labs, the vaccine would be manufactured. Depending upon the availability, the at-risk population would be prioritized for vaccination.

(iii) Non-Pharmaceutical Intervention

The non-pharmaceutical intervention would include measures that need to be instituted at individual, community and national level.

At **individual** level there would be isolation of the patient and quarantine of those exposed. Individuals should follow simple public health measures for infection control such as hand washing, respiratory etiquettes, staying away from those having respiratory symptoms and by using masks. At this level, self recognition of illness and self reporting to identified health facility would be encouraged.

At the **community** level, during phase 5/6, community wide quarantine (restricting entry/ exit of population from a defined geographic area) is only advocated if the virus is not efficiently transmitting, mass chemoprophylaxis could be achieved and resources are available to implement and maintain quarantine. Essential services also need to be ensured with in the quarantined community.

For phase 5/6, social distancing measures need to be imposed such as closure of school, college, business, cinemas, theatres and markets. School closure is especially useful if high morbidity among children is seen and should be implemented early. Mass gatherings such as festivals, weekly markets, sporting events, religious and social congregations, funerals etc need to be discouraged or cancelled. Public transportation need to be restricted and should also be achieved by voluntary or involuntary work holidays.

At the **national level**, Indian citizens would be advised to defer non essential travel. Information would be provided to travelers regarding the disease. Entry screening would be imposed at all international airports, ports and international checkpoints. If India got affected with community outbreaks, then exit screening would be considered.

(iv) Medical Care

Until such time that India is not having any clusters, the entry screening would be complimented by dedicated isolation facilities where the suspect cases could be kept. The preparedness measures to be put in place for phase 6 would see health workers trained on triage and referral and providing domestic care.

The CRB-65 clinical assessment tool would be adopted. Hospital disaster manual would have provisions for surge capacity. It should address emergency staffing needs and increased demand for isolation wards, ICUs, ventilatory management and the logistic support required for these. If need be, patients could be accommodated in temporary hospitals.

Defence (especially for Cantonment Board area), Railways and Employees State Insurance Corporation (ESI) have a number of hospitals. These organizations would contribute towards the surge capacity.

The private sector, which caters to over 70 per cent of the medical needs of the country would also be made to contribute to provide health care on an equitable basis.

(v) Risk Communication

Risk Communication would be the most important non-pharmaceutical intervention. The risk and risk reduction strategies/actions would be communicated in clear consistent messages and widely disseminated through print and visual media.

Institutional Framework

Inter-sectoral coordination is essence of managing pandemic. As the pandemic phase changes from phase three to six, substantial role is envisaged for sectors other than health. Ultimately for managing phase 6 of the pandemic, the activities have to be dovetailed into the disaster management frame work. The foregoing paragraphs identify mechanism for the sectoral co-ordination, the institutional mechanism at national, state and district level and define their roles and responsibilities.

(a) National Level

The National Disaster Management Authority and National Crisis Management Committee would review the preparedness and response and issue strategic directions for the containment operations/mitigation measures.

Inter Ministerial Task Force

Policy decisions and inter sectoral issues would be decided in the Inter Ministerial Task Force. The constitution of the Task Force is as under:

Secretary (Health & FW)	— Chairman
Secretary (Animal Husbandry)	— Member
Secretary (Information and Broad casting)	— Member
Secretary (Civil aviation)	— Member
Secretary (Home)	— Member
Secretary (Chemicals and Fertilisers)	— Member
Secretary (Defence)	— Member
Secretary (NDMA)	— Member
Secretary and DG, ICMR	— Member
Director General of Health Services	— Member
Special DGHS (Public Health)	— Member
Mission Director, NRHM	— Member
Additional Secretary (H&FW)	— Member Secretary

The Task Force would co-opt members from other sectors as required.

Joint Monitoring Group

The Joint Monitoring Group would recommend on technical matters and monitor outbreak situation. The constitution of the Joint Monitoring Group is:

Director General of Health Services	— Chairman
DG, ICMR	— Member
Special DGHS	— Member
Animal Husbandry Commissioner	— Member
Representative of M/o Home Ministry	— Member
Representative of M/o I&B	— Member
Representative of M/o Environment and Forest	— Member
Sr DDG, ICMR	— Member
Representative NDMA	— Member
HoD, Respiratory Medicine, AIIMS	— Member
HoD, Microbiology, AIIMS	— Member
HoD, Epidemiology, NICD	— Member
HoD, Microbiology, NICD	— Member
WR,WHO	— Member
Director (EMR)	— Member Secretary

The institutions as well as their individual role and responsibilities are:

Ministry of Health and Family Welfare (MOHFW)

Ministry of Health and Family Welfare (MOHFW) would be the nodal ministry. It would support States in managing human cases caused by a novel influenza virus. The participating units would be:

- Public Health Division, MOHFW.
- Emergency Medical Relief (EMR) Division of Directorate General of Health Services (Dte GHS), MOHFW.
- International Health Division, Dte GHS, MOHFW.
- National Institute of Communicable Diseases (NICD) and Integrated Disease Surveillance Project.
- Central Government Hospitals.
- Institutions under Indian Council of Medical Research (ICMR).

MOHFW will be supported by other ministries such as Home Affairs, Agriculture, Civil Aviation, Defence, External Affairs, Information and Broadcasting, Chemicals and Fertilizers and other ministries as deemed relevant for the management operations.

MOHFW will also liaison with the international agencies namely WHO (technical and logistic support) and UNICEF (IEC etc).

Ministry of Home Affairs (MHA)

MHA would facilitate:

- Border control to prevent cross border spread.
- Augmenting state security forces for facilitating perimeter control of containment zone for restricting movement of human population.
- Support the state in maintaining law and order.
- Provide support for restriction of movement in and from the affected area.
- Enforcing social distancing measures.
- Provide support for airlift of RRTs/logistics/samples to and from inaccessible areas.

Ministry of External Affairs (MEA)

- Liaison with affected countries, arranging bi-lateral or multi lateral meetings.
- Raising issues in international and regional forums.
- Visa restriction, if required.
- Providing information on foreign nationals travelling to India.

Ministry of Defence

- Training faculty of its medical colleges and cantonment hospitals and Station Health Officers on pandemic preparedness and response.
- Extend hospital services, especially in cantonment areas to civilians.
- Provide research support to ICMR.

Ministry of Railways

- Train doctors in railway hospitals on pandemic preparedness and response.
- Extend hospital services to civilians.
- Transportation of medical supplies

Ministry of Civil Aviation

- Provide support for airlift of RRT/logistics/samples.
- Facilitate exit screening/entry screening.
- Provide the screening proforma to the airlines.
- Provide space for screening, clinical examination and quarantine.
- Provide space for setting up of Airport Health Organization.

Ministry of Shipping, Surface Transport and Highways

- Facilitate exit screening/entry screening
- Port Quarantine
- Restriction of public transport.

Ministry of Consumer Affairs, Food and Public Distribution

- Maintain essential food supply to the Quarantine area
- Maintain essential food supply during pandemic phase.

Ministry of Information and Broadcasting

- Develop Media strategy
- Role out appropriate communication materials for National and State campaign.
- Facilitate availability of slots for media communication in print/visual media.
- Utilize the field publicity units for social mobilization.

Ministry of Agriculture (Department of Animal Husbandry)

- Provide information on unusual poultry deaths to MOHFW at the earliest but not later than 24 hours (if concurrent outbreaks are taking place among poultry).
- Convey the laboratory test results of the poultry deaths at the earliest.
- Keep close liaison with MOHFW, especially if the human cluster has happened an area where poultry outbreak is ongoing/has been reported/post operation surveillance activities are continuing.

National Disaster Management Authority (NDMA)

NDMA would co-ordinate integration of Pandemic influenza prevention, preparedness and response with existing disaster management frame work at all levels. This would include a co-ordinated mechanism for health and sectors beyond health for maintaining essential services and continuity of operations. Also such co-ordination mechanism would be established between Government and non-government entities. The plans of all critical sectors would be approved by NDMA and implementation monitored.

NDMA would monitor the progress of the pandemic and the impact of the mitigation measures in health and sectors other than health.

(b) State Level

Chief Secretary would ensure co-ordination between health, home and other relevant departments. The State would sensitize administrators on pandemic and actions to be taken in health and sectors beyond health.

The Principal Secretary/Secretary of the State Health Department will take administrative and financial decisions with regard to prevention, preparedness and response activities pertaining to the health sector. A Technical Committee under DHS would provide the technical support.

The State Health Department would draw up its pandemic plan and test it. The plan would provide for surveillance for detecting cases early, institute preparedness measures, provide training to State and District RRTs, stock personal protective equipments and provide necessary infrastructure for clinical management of cases. Health workers would be trained on triage and clinical management.

The Central Government's efforts in creating awareness among the community on mitigating the risks would be further facilitated by the State's own initiatives through both print and visual media.

State Disaster Management Authority (SDMA)

SDMA would co-ordinate integration of Pandemic Influenza prevention, preparedness and response with existing disaster management frame work at State level. This would include a co-ordinated mechanism of health and sectors beyond health for maintaining essential services and continuity of operations in States and districts.

Such co-ordination mechanism would be established between Government and Non-Government entities. The District plans of all would be approved by SDMA and implementation monitored.

(c) District Level

District Collector would assume charge of overall co-ordination. The Chief Medical Officer would support in implementing all actions pertaining to health sector. The District IDSP would be responsible for surveillance for ILI and pneumonia cases. The District Rapid Response Team would investigate the outbreak and provide support in instituting public health measures.

In phase-6, the District Disaster Management Authority would be responsible for all actions for sectors other than health. The institution of the containment/ mitigation measures and maintaining essential services would be done by the district machinery through the grass root level functionaries.

Essential Capacities

The essential capacities for each component will vary and will not all be present in every Member State. The capacity to detect, assess, respond to, and report public health emergencies of international concern, which relates to the first component of pandemic surveillance, is mandated by International Health Regulations for all Member States. In addition, the ability to do adequate case investigations and routine monitoring of respiratory disease activity is a capacity that has value beyond the evaluation and monitoring of influenza virus with pandemic potential. Specific capacities for each component of surveillance include:

Early Detection and Investigation

- A system able to detect and report events that are a potential risk to public health.
- Laboratory capacity to identify influenza viruses with pandemic potential or rapid access to outside laboratory facilities with this capacity.
- Epidemiological expertise to carry out the initial investigation of signal events.
- A national IHR focal point to report public health emergencies of international concern to WHO.
- Outbreak response and pandemic preparedness plans.
- Materials and personnel for rapid containment of outbreaks of influenza with pandemic potential.

Comprehensive Assessment

- Laboratory capacity or access to laboratory capacity for virus culture, polymerase chain reaction (PCR), and serological testing.
- Epidemiological capacity for extended field investigation and detailed analysis of case data.
- Supplies and personnel for a large field investigation

involving hundreds of potential cases and contact tracing.

- Communications and data transfer capability.

Monitoring

- Routine surveillance for influenza-like illness (ILI) and/or severe acute respiratory illness (SARI).
- Epidemiological capacity for data analysis and interpretation.
- Communication systems for regular reporting of surveillance data internationally.

Action Plan

Early Detection and Investigation

Key Points

- *Goal:* Detect and confirm sustained human-to-human transmission of an influenza virus with pandemic potential or start of the pandemic.
- *Reporting:* Through the National IHR Focal Point to the WHO IHR Contact Point and including the WHO Country Office where applicable:
  - First affected country: Complete Case Summary Forms and report of investigation.
  - Subsequently infected countries: Report first appearance of pandemic virus.
- *Benefits for affected Member State:* Joint risk assessment with WHO, data will inform containment efforts, WHO support in risk communications.
- *Benefit at global level:* Other Members States are alerted on basis of official data.

Comprehensive Assessment

Key Points

- *Goal:* Provide accurate description of epidemiological, clinical and virological characteristics of the emerging pandemic.
- *Reporting:*

  - Epidemiological data
  - Clinical data
  - Virological characteristics
  - Investigation methods.
- *Benefit for Member States:* Assess the severity of the event and guide national control activities.
- *Benefit at global level:* Inform pandemic vaccine composition; provide early assessment of severity; - update response plans and tailor control measures to the severity of the event.

Monitoring

Key Points

- *Goal:* Track the course of the pandemic.
- *Reporting:*
  - Activity
  - Geographic spread
  - Trend
  - Intensity
  - Impact on health care system
  - Quantitative data on cases and deaths of ILI and/or SARI if possible
- *Benefit for Member States:* Modify mitigation and management strategies in response to changes in the course of the pandemic.
- *Benefit at global level:* Decide on changes in pandemic phase; anticipate second wave.

Early Detection and Investigation

Launch investigation for evidence of sustained human-to-human transmission

Refine case management and control measures:

- Estimate geographic extent
- Alert Member States
- Track activity
- Track geographical spread
- Track trend of pandemic

- Track impact of pandemic
  Adjust allocation of health care resources, initiate additional management strategies as indicated
- Track intensity of transmission
  Monitor changes in antigenicity and antiviral sensitivity
  Adjust use of pharmaceutical interventions

Partnering with Media to Combat Pandemic Influenza

The Ministry of Health & Family Welfare joined hands with WHO, UNICEF and the media to strategize on how to inform and protect the public from Pandemic H1N1 (2009) Influenza at the National Media Communication Workshop held in New Delhi on 23-24 July, 2009.

The key is not having a plan in place, but actually implementing and executing the plan. The plan that has been designed seems to 'hitting the nail on the head'; but unfortunately, owing to the factors listed below, it has not been executed as planned:

- Inadequate interdepartmental communication within the administration
- Inadequate communication between health authorities and administration
- Inadequate communication and guidelines provided to the media to act as a tool for spreading awareness
- Lack of 'preparedness' on part of the medical authorities
- Availability of the basic safety equipments such as 'masks' in the black market

Thus, the basic requirement is having a system in place which can efficiently execute all the plans; a team of individuals who are dedicated towards ensuring the health of the denizens of the country.

The importance of efficiency cannot be undermined, simply because it is the one factor which would ensure that the disease is contained as far along as possible. It would also help save time; and this being a race against time to bring about containment, it would prove to be some solace if we could do that!

CHAPTER 9

International Guidelines to Mitigate the Pandemic

The Public Health Agency of Canada announced that their National Microbiology Laboratory (NML) had mapped the genetic code of the swine flu virus, the first time that was done.

U.S officials noted that six years of worrying about H5N1 avian flu did much to prepare for the current swine flu outbreak, noting that after H5N1 emerged widely in Asia in 2003, killing about 60 percent of the humans infected by it, many countries took steps to prevent any similar crisis.

Contingency Planning

Although most flu symptoms are mild and last only a few days without treatment, health officials worldwide are concerned because the virus is new and could easily mutate and become more virulent.

To combat the virus, WHO and the U.S. government are gearing up for a massive vaccination campaign later this year, one not seen since Jonas Salk discovered the polio vaccine in 1955 and it was made available worldwide.

Officials are also urging communities, businesses and individuals to make contingency plans for possible school closures, multiple employee absences for illness, surges of patients in hospitals and other effects of potentially widespread outbreaks. It is estimated that as many as 40% of the workforce, in a worst-case scenario, might be unable to work at the peak of the pandemic due to the need for many healthy adults to stay home and care for an ill family member. This implies that they need to thin ahead and have a back-up plan in place to be able to cope with such a situation.

An opinion article by specialist Eric Toner in the *New York Times* notes that if the 2009 flu follows patterns from earlier pandemics, the U.S. may experience a much bigger, second wave of the pandemic early in the fall, perhaps before a vaccine is widely available, and advised preparations to avoid crowding of hospital emergency departments.

It suggests that patients with mild symptoms should be told that flu can usually be treated by home care with rest, fluids, and acetaminophen and ibuprofen for fever, while suggesting alternative treatment options including extended physician and clinic hours and special flu clinics run by volunteers.

It advised hospitals to cancel vacations, reassign personnel, require mandatory overtime, and to pool resources and patient loads.

Schools

Schools and universities worldwide have been on alert and working with health officials to launch education campaigns. Many plan to stockpile medical supplies and discuss worst-case scenarios, including plans to provide lessons and meals for low-income children in case elementary and secondary schools close.

To help prepare for contingencies, some medical experts in the U.S. suggest that every county should create an "influenza action team" to be run by the local health department, parents, and school administrators.

There have been instances of schools getting closed for sometime, but they are seen as unnecessary, as the virus spreads far too quickly for this particular step to have any reasonable effect.

Instead, the CDC recommends that students and school workers with flu symptoms should stay home for seven days, and those who are sick longer should not come back to school until 24 hours after symptoms subside.

Airlines

The president of the Association of Flight Attendants told members of a U.S. Congressional subcommittee that all flight attendants should be given training in how to handle a person with flu and help in communicating to passengers the importance of keeping clean hands, and that flight attendants need to be provided gloves and facemasks to deal with flu-stricken passengers.

Other medical experts add that airlines should also ensure that passenger cabins are always properly ventilated, including during any flight delays in which passengers are kept aboard the plane. But they also add that although the aviation industry in the U.S., along with the CDC, have tried to reassure passengers that air travel is safe, they have so far done too little to try to limit infection risks.

Travel Advisories

The new strain has spread widely beyond North America with confirmed cases in eighty-nine countries. Initially, most cases outside North America were following recent travel to Mexico or the U.S. However by May 15 in-country transmission had been reported from Canada, Japan, Panama, the UK, Spain, Germany, Australia, Italy, and Belgium, and as of June 17 most countries within the European Union had documented in-country transmission, as had many countries worldwide.

Many countries had earlier advised citizens to avoid travelling to infected areas and were monitoring visitors returning from flu-affected areas for flu symptoms.

WHO guidance from 7 May recommends no travel restrictions based on this strain of influenza stating that scientific research based on mathematical modelling shows that restricting travel would be of limited or no benefit in stopping the spread of disease.

The CDC downgraded a previous "Travel Health Warning" for Mexico to a "Travel Health Precaution" on May 15 referring to the reduction in infections in Mexico and the reduced overall risk of the virus.

Actions Concerning Pigs

International health officials have reaffirmed that pork is safe to eat and hogs are not to blame for the epidemic. However, as of early June, China, Russia and more than a dozen other countries were still banning pork imports from the U.S.

The World Trade Organisation (WTO) planned to highlight the pork bans in a forthcoming report on protectionism and reiterate that cooked pork is not a source of infection and is safe to eat.

In June, the U.S. Agriculture Department said it would launch a pilot surveillance project to look for new strains of flu virus in pigs. Some experts claim that global health officials have underestimated the risk that pig herds might be a source of new influenza strains but have instead focused on the threat of bird flu.

Travel Alerts to the People's Republic of China

In late May 2009, the Chinese government confined 21 U.S. students and three teachers to their hotel rooms because a passenger on their plane to People's Republic of China, suspected of having swine flu, had been seated within four rows of the students.

As a result, on June 22, the U.S. State Department issued a travel alert about China's anti-flu measures, and is warning travellers that PR China is imposing the seven-day quarantine on passengers arriving with a fever or flu-like symptoms in order to prevent the flu spreading in the country.

The US State Department also said it had received reports about unsuitable quarantine conditions, including the unavailability of suitable drinking water and food, unsanitary conditions, and the inability to communicate with others.

All travelers to China, including U.S. citizens, are obliged to follow local public health-related measures, and there is no compensation for lost travel expenses. Travellers to China should consider buying travel insurance to protect against losses in case they are quarantined, recommended the State Department.

Other Government Quarantines

Other governments have taken or threatened similar quarantine actions: In **Hong Kong**, an entire hotel was quarantined with 240 guests after one person staying there was found to have swine flu.

The government of **Australia** ordered a cruise ship with 2000 passengers to stay at sea because of a swine flu threat.

Egyptians who went on the annual Muslim pilgrimage to Mecca risked being quarantined upon their return. Also, a foreign students' dormitory for the American University in Cairo, with 140 students, was put under quarantine after two U.S. students were diagnosed with swine flu.

At the end of April 2009, when the outbreak began, **Russia** and **Taiwan** said they would quarantine visitors showing symptoms of the virus.

In **Southern California**, a marine confirmed to have swine flu was placed in quarantine along with about 30 other Marines.

In early May, **Japan** quarantined 47 airline passengers in a hotel for a week after three travelers who arrived on the same plane from Canada tested positive for H1N1 swine flu.

Mongolia quarantined 109 Russian airline passengers in Ulaanbator.

In **India**, after four airline passengers from London tested positive, the government ordered that all the 231 passengers of the flight should be administered the anti viral drug oseltamivir. Health authorities also asked that all the passengers not move out of their homes until further orders and quarantined at least one of the infected passengers.

Other governments have given health officials the "increased power" to order people into quarantine to control the spread of swine flu. The government of **New Zealand,** for instance, gave medical officers the power to order people to be quarantined at home if they have been in close contact with someone who had swine flu.

Pre-Screening Advisories by Some Governments

Some governments have also suggested pre-screening "outbound" passengers from countries that are thought to have a high rate of infection. India's Minister of State for Health, for example, said on June 16, that there should be "some kind of screening" for outbound travellers in the U.S., claiming that most people coming from that country have been tested positive for influenza A(H1N1) virus.

Spread in the Workplace

The CDC advised sick people to stay home from work, school, or social gatherings and to generally limit contact with others to avoid infecting them.

In the UK, the HSE has also issued general guidance for employers.

Emergency Planning

Emergency preparedness experts suggest that organizations, such as corporations, should be making plans now in case something big and unexpected happens with the Swine Flu or other potential pandemic viruses.

This would include some of the following:

- Asking people with symptoms, and members of an ill person's household, to voluntarily remain at home for up to 7 days.
- Sending students home from school, including public and private schools as well as colleges and universities, and recommending out-of-school social distancing.
- Recommending social distancing of adults which could include cancelling public gatherings or changing workplace environment.

Crime Risk

In early June, the Australian Crime Commission, in a written public report, warned that criminals may exploit a swine flu pandemic. They pointed out that illicit markets, robbery and fraud through false charities were all potential targets for organised crime, and the emergence of a black market for medicine was also a concern.

It warns of potential robbery and extortion, counterfeit medicine scams, black markets, charity fraud, welfare fraud and possibly increased community influence. Industrial drug sites might be targeted for robbery along with retail chemists.

During a polio outbreak in 1959, for instance, masked bandits stole 75,000 Salk vaccine shots from a Montreal university research center.

In late May, the U.S. Food and Drug Administration (FDA) uncovered spurious swine flu treatments available on the Internet. They have reportedly ordered dozens of Web site operators to stop making fraudulent claims.

In the six weeks since FDA's campaign began the number of new sites selling fake swine flu treatments and protective devices has plummeted, whereas at the beginning they were seeing as many as 10 new Web sites a day selling fraudulent products.

In India too, amidst growing concerns, private chemists have been selling face masks at exorbitant prices, and have reportedly been threats of the drug Tamiflu having been stolen in some quantities.

Ministry of Health and Family Welfare, Government of India

Guidelines for Schools/Colleges/Institutions on Influenza A H1N1

There have been some cases of Influenza A H1N1 virus among students and staff in certain schools, primarily in Delhi and Maharashtra. There has been considerable speculation over the need for closure of schools to control the outbreak. This matter has been considered by the Joint Monitoring Group in the Ministry of Health and Family Welfare. All schools and colleges are advised to observe the following guidelines for managing cases of infection of Influenza A H1N1:

- Any student or staff member showing flu like symptoms such as fever, cough, running nose and difficulty in breathing should be allowed to stay at home for a period of 7 to 10 days.
- Educational institutions should not insist on production of medical certificate by the student/staff.
- Educational institutions should monitor the health status of such students/staff who might have come in contact with a suspected case of Influenza AH1N1 to see whether they develop flu like symptoms.

In case they do so, they should be allowed to stay home, as outlined above

- In case of students staying in hostels, the educational institutions would not only monitor the health status of the students, but also that of care providers.
- It has to be ensured that the care providers wear face mask and wash hands regularly. It might not be advisable to send the boarders back to home, as it would spread infection further.
- Educational institutions are further encouraged to report such cases to local health officers for further monitoring.
- Given the current magnitude of the spread of AH1N1 infection and the fact that the current virus is fairly mild, closure of educational institutions on account of any student/staff member falling ill with flu like symptoms is not recommended.
- In the first place, the schools should discourage the excursions of the students to the affectedcountries.
- In case if the students had proceeded to affected countries on unavoidable tours, then on their return, if some students show flu like symptoms of fever, sore- throat , cough , body ache, running nose, difficulty breathing etc. they should be advised to abstain from attending school and be allowed to stay at home for a period of 7 to 10 days.

Revised Guidelines for testing of persons with flu like symptoms reporting at hospitals notified for Influenza A H1N1

So far, the present guidelines stipulate that a person suspected of influenza A H1N1 need to be referred to an identified govt. health facility. He/she needs to be kept in an isolation facility in that hospital and if found positive, is treated accordingly.

In order to make the testing facility for H1N1 more accessible at large and due to the onset of the Influenza season in the country, it has been decided to revise the existing guidelines.

Under the new guidelines:

- Any person with flu like symptoms such as fever, cough, sore throat, cold, running nose etc. should go to a designated Government facility for giving his/her sample for testing for the H1N1 virus. After clinical assessment, the designated medical officer would decide on the need for testing. Except for cases that are severe, the patient would be allowed to go home (This was not allowed under the existing guidelines).
- The sample of the suspect case would be collected and sent to the notified laboratory for testing. If tested as positive for H1N1 and in case the symptoms are mild, the patient would be informed and given the option of admission into the hospital or isolation and treatment at his own home.
- In case the patient opts for home isolation and treatment, he/she would be provided with detailed guidelines/ safety measures to be strictly adhered to by the entire household of the patient. He/she would have to provide full contact details of his entire household. The house hold and social contacts would be provided with the preventive treatment.
- Notwithstanding the above guidelines, the decision of the doctor of the notified hospital about admitting the patient would be final.
- In case the test is negative, the patient will accordingly be informed.

These guidelines have been issued by the Government in public interest and shall be reviewed from time to time depending on the spread of the pandemic and its severity in the country.

These guidelines would however not apply to passengers who are identified through screening at the points of entry. The existing policy of isolating passengers with flu like symptoms would continue.

CHAPTER 10

What Lies Ahead

To a naturalist, it is no surprise that these viruses keep coming back, much more potent, and always able to evade the means tha we have crreated to keep them at bay. It is nothing but evolution; a law of nature: survival of the fittest.

Nature does not discriminate between her different creations. She selects randomly; without ever being biased. So what was nothing but a chunk of organic matter became a single cell, which eventually proliferated and diverged into all that we know as life. Also, some went retrogade evolution and disappeared, or became semiautonomous; like the chloroplasts in plants, or the mitochondria in all living cells.

Parallelly, along this road to evolution, there were lost a few genes here and there, which gradually came together and made enough sense of their aggregation to be able to survive in living cells. These were the first viruses. Or they could also be vestigial quasi-living organisms of the aeons gone by.

Whatever their course, in the modern era, viruses are seen as big threats to health, (and some would say even wealth) of nations worldwide. They are difficult to control and eradicate. Many of the animal viruses have very peculiar mechanisms of replication and unusually, their genetic material is RNA, instead of DNA.

Why RNA when DNA was chosen by evolution to be the genetic material of choice? could these be primitive organisms?

It would be a huge mistake to undermine their significance. Perhaps their genetic material being RNA is not as stable as DNA, but they have made another deal with nature; instead of stability, they have used the instability of their genomes to their advantage.

Many RNA viruses have short generation times and relatively high mutation rates (on the order of one point mutation or more per genome per round of replication for RNA viruses). This elevated mutation rate, when combined with natural selection, allows viruses to quickly adapt to changes in their host environment.

The high error rate inherent in all RNA synthesis provides RNA virus genomes with extremely high mutation rates. Thus nearly all large RNA virus clonal populations are *quasispecies* collections of differing, related genomes. These rapidly mutating populations can remain remarkably stable under certain conditions of replication.

Under other conditions, virus-population equilibria become disturbed, and extremely rapid evolution can result. This is an important aspect of the epidemiology of viral diseases such as influenza (Influenza virus), AIDS (HIV), and hepatitis (e.g. HCV). It presents daunting challenges for the design of effective vaccines for the control of diseases caused by rapidly evolving RNA virus populations.It also causes problems in the development of successful vaccines and antiviral drugs, as resistant mutations often appear within weeks or months after the beginning of the treatment.

Quasispecies Model

The **quasispecies model** is a description of the process of the Darwinian evolution of certain self-replicating entities within the framework of physical chemistry. Put simply, a quasispecies is a large group or **cloud** of related genotypes that exist in an environment of high mutation rate, where a large fraction of offspring are expected to contain one or more mutations relative to the parent. This is in contrast to a species, which from an evolutionary perspective is a more-or-less stable single genotype, most of the offspring of which will be genetically accurate copies.

It is useful mainly in providing a qualitative understanding of the evolutionary processes of self-replicating macromolecules such as RNA or DNA or simple asexual organisms such as bacteria or viruses, and is helpful in explaining something of the early stages of the origin of life. Quantitative predictions based on this model are difficult because the parameters that serve as its input are hard to obtain from actual biological systems.

In a species, though reproduction may be mostly accurate, periodic mutations will give rise to one or more competing genotypes. If a mutation results in greater replication and survival, the mutant genotype may out-compete the parent genotype and come to dominate the species. Thus, the individual genotypes (or species) may be seen as the units on which selection acts and biologists will often speak of a single genotype's fitness.

In a quasispecies, however, mutations are ubiquitous and so the fitness of an individual genotype becomes meaningless: if one particular mutation generates a boost in reproductive success it can't amount to much because that genotype's offspring are unlikely to be accurate copies with the same properties. Instead, what matters is the *connectedness* of the cloud.

The analogue of fitness for a quasispecies is the tendency of nearby relatives within the cloud to be well-connected, meaning that more of the mutant descendants will be viable and give rise to further descendants within the cloud.

The model rests on four assumptions:

1. The self-replicating entities can be represented as sequences composed of a small number of building blocks—for example, sequences of RNA consisting of the four bases adenine, guanine, cytosine, and uracil.
2. New sequences enter the system solely as the result of a copy process, either correct or erroneous, of other sequences that are already present.
3. The substrates, or raw materials, necessary for ongoing replication are always present in sufficient quantity. Excess sequences are washed away in an outgoing flux.
4. Sequences may decay into their building blocks. The

probability of decay does not depend on the sequences' age; old sequences are just as likely to decay as young sequences.

In the quasispecies model, mutations occur through errors made in the process of copying already existing sequences. Further, selection arises because different types of sequences tend to replicate at different rates, which leads to the suppression of sequences that replicate more slowly in favor of sequences that replicate faster.

However, the quasispecies model does not predict the ultimate extinction of all but the fastest replicating sequence. Although the sequences that replicate more slowly cannot sustain their abundance level by themselves, they are constantly replenished as sequences that replicate faster mutate into them. At equilibrium, removal of slowly replicating sequences due to decay or outflow is balanced by replenishing, so that even relatively slowly replicating sequences can remain present in finite abundance.

Due to the ongoing production of mutant sequences, selection does not act on single sequences, but on mutational "clouds" of closely related sequences, referred to as *quasispecies*. In other words, the evolutionary success of a particular sequence depends not only on its own replication rate, but also on the replication rates of the mutant sequences it produces, and on the replication rates of the sequences of which it is a mutant. As a consequence, the sequence that replicates fastest may even disappear completely in selection-mutation equilibrium, in favor of more slowly replicating sequences that are part of a quasispecies with a higher average growth rate. Mutational clouds as predicted by the quasispecies model have been observed in RNA viruses and in *in vitro* RNA replication.

The mutation rate and the general fitness of the molecular sequences and their neighbors is crucial to the formation of a quasispecies. If the mutation rate is zero, there is no exchange by mutation, and each sequence is its own species. If the mutation rate is too high, exceeding what is known as the error threshold, the quasispecies will break down and be dispersed over the entire range of available sequences.

The Implications of Gene Technology

Modern gene technology, as we know it, has proved to be a whole new world when it comes to understanding ourselves, and the orders that govern us. However, it could prove to be a handful when dealing with the experiments that we have come to love performing.

Whether it be sequencing a genome, which gives access to the genetic structure of the most potent organisms and the ease of access of such sensitive information to all, or recombinant DNA technology, which allows us to fiddle with nature; all these could prove to be a bane with the slightest mishandling.

There have been numerous fears of using H1N1 as a weapon for bioterrorism afetr its etire genome was published in *Science* after sequencing. All Influenza A pandemics since the Spanish Flu pandemic, and indeed almost all cases of influenza A worldwide (excepting human infections from avian viruses such as H5N1 and H7N7), have been caused by descendants of the 1918 virus, including "drifted" H1N1 viruses and reassorted H2N2 and H3N2 viruses. The latter are composed of key genes from the 1918 virus, updated by subsequently incorporated avian influenza genes that code for novel surface proteins, making the 1918 virus indeed the "mother" of all pandemics.

Thus sequencing the genomes of such potent organisms can allow anti-social elements to use this as an opportunity to create new waves of terror, thereby proving that uncontrolled and unrestricted use of technology has its downfalls.

We have already had a glimpse of it when post 9/11, the FBI received letters containing cultured spores of *Bacillus anthracis*, the bacteria causing anthrax.

Technology in the wrong hands is not the only worry though. It is after fifty years of creating plastics that we have realised what a menace they are for the environment. Suppose a recombinant experiment goes wrong and empowers a potentially latent organism, or one with a weakened virulence. The consequences of such an act will not take fifty years to be seen; amidst all concerns around us, this could then take centre stage.

Thus, the future with regards the evolution of viruses can never be ascertained. It is very hard to say when or where will a new strain of virus emerge which can cause lethal outbreaks, epidemics or pandemics. It is even more difficult in present circumstances with so many experiments that we are trying to carry out with the nature of life; for we might unwittingly give them an advantage which would make competing amongst a myriad of organisms much easier, and life for us much more difficult.

And so, while we are looking at empowering our understanding of nature to the very elements that have come together to create life, we should also remember that no matter how hard we try, we will still always be just a part of this kaleidoscope of life; not the centre of life itself.

We must be grateful that nature has given us the intelligence to understand and appreciate her creations, but it is nature which has the power to control them. if we try to shift the centre of power, we might get something thrown at us from her which could prove cataclysmic to our very existence.

CHAPTER 11

Frequently Asked Questions

Owing to the growing panic among the people, there have been numerous enquiries with regards the H1N1 Influenza. Since it has been unknown, there are many myths and misnomers that people have about the diseases.

In the following section, we aim to correct those misnomers and further the readers' knowledge about the disease.

Novel H1N1 Flu

(1) What is novel H1N1 (swine flu)?

Novel H1N1 (referred to as "swine flu" early on) is a new influenza virus causing illness in people. This new virus was first detected in people in the United States in April 2009. This virus is spreading from person-to-person worldwide, probably in much the same way that regular seasonal influenza viruses spread. On June 11, 2009, the World Health Organization (WHO) signaled that a pandemic of novel H1N1 flu was underway.

(2) Why is novel H1N1 virus sometimes called "swine flu"?

This virus was originally referred to as "swine flu" because laboratory testing showed that many of the genes in this new virus were very similar to influenza viruses that normally occur in pigs (swine) in North America. But further study has shown that this new virus is very different from what normally circulates in North American pigs. It has two genes from flu viruses that normally circulate in pigs in Europe and Asia and bird (avian) genes and human genes. Scientists call this a "quadruple reassortant" virus.

(3) **How many H1N1 (swine) flu viruses are there?**

Like all influenza viruses, swine flu viruses change constantly. Pigs can be infected by avian influenza and human influenza viruses as well as swine influenza viruses. When influenza viruses from different species infect pigs, the viruses can reassort (i.e. swap genes) and new viruses that are a mix of swine, human and/or avian influenza viruses can emerge. Over the years, different variations of swine flu viruses have emerged. At this time, there are four main influenza type A virus subtypes that have been isolated in pigs: H1N1, H1N2, H3N2, and H3N1. However, most of the recently isolated influenza viruses from pigs have been H1N1 viruses.

Novel H1N1 Flu in Humans

(4) **Are there human infections with novel H1N1 virus?**

Yes. Human infections with the new H1N1 virus are ongoing all around the world. Most people who have become ill with this new virus have recovered without requiring medical treatment. CDC routinely works with states to collect, compile and analyze information about influenza, and has done the same for the new H1N1 virus since the beginning of the outbreak.

(5) **Is novel H1N1 virus contagious?**

CDC has determined that novel H1N1 virus is contagious and is spreading from human to human.

(6) **How does novel H1N1 virus spread?**

Spread of novel H1N1 virus is thought to occur in the same way that seasonal flu spreads. Flu viruses are spread mainly from person to person through coughing or sneezing by people with influenza. Sometimes people may become infected by touching something – such as a surface or object – with flu viruses on it and then touching their mouth or nose.

(7) **What are the signs and symptoms of this virus in people?**

The symptoms of novel H1N1 flu virus in people include fever, cough, sore throat, runny or stuffy nose, body aches, headache, chills and fatigue. A significant number of people who have been infected with this virus also have reported diarrhea and vomiting. Severe illnesses and death has occurred as a result of illness associated with this virus.

(8) **How severe is illness associated with novel H1N1 flu virus?**

Illness with the new H1N1 virus has ranged from mild to severe. While most people who have been sick have recovered without needing medical treatment, hospitalizations and deaths from infection with this virus have occurred.

In seasonal flu, certain people are at "high risk" of serious complications. This includes people 65 years and older, children younger than five years old, pregnant women, and people of any age with certain chronic medical conditions. About 70 percent of people who have been hospitalized with this novel H1N1 virus have had one or more medical conditions previously recognized as placing people at "high risk" of serious seasonal flu-related complications. This includes pregnancy, diabetes, heart disease, asthma and kidney disease.

(9) **How does novel H1N1 flu compare to seasonal flu in terms of its severity and infection rates?**

With seasonal flu, we know that seasons vary in terms of timing, duration and severity. Seasonal influenza can cause mild to severe illness, and at times can lead to death. Each year, in the United States, on average 36,000 people die from flu-related complications and more than 200,000 people are hospitalized from flu-related causes. Of those hospitalized, 20,000 are children younger than 5 years old. Over 90% of deaths and about 60 percent of hospitalization occur in people older than 65.

When the novel H1N1 outbreak was first detected in mid-April 2009, CDC began working with states to collect, compile and analyze information regarding the novel H1N1 flu outbreak, including the numbers of confirmed and probable cases and the ages of these people. The information analyzed by CDC supports the conclusion that novel H1N1 flu has caused greater disease burden in people younger than 25 years of age than older people. At this time, there are few cases and few deaths reported in people older than 64 years old, which is unusual when compared with seasonal flu. However, pregnancy and other previously recognized high risk medical conditions from seasonal influenza appear to be associated with increased risk of complications from this novel H1N1. These underlying conditions include asthma, diabetes, suppressed immune systems, heart disease, kidney disease, neurocognitive and neuromuscular disorders and pregnancy.

(10) How long can an infected person spread this virus to others?

People infected with seasonal and novel H1N1 flu shed virus and may be able to infect others from 1 day before getting sick to 5 to 7 days after. This can be longer in some people, especially children and people with weakened immune systems and in people infected with the new H1N1 virus.

Prevention and Treatment

(11) What can I do to protect myself from getting sick?

There is no vaccine available right now to protect against novel H1N1 virus. However, a novel H1N1 vaccine is currently in production and may be ready for the public in the fall.

There are everyday actions that can help prevent the spread of germs that cause respiratory illnesses like influenza involving basic hygience and cleanliness, along with avoiding crowded areas.

Other important actions that you can take are:

- Follow public health advice regarding school closures, avoiding crowds and other social distancing measures.
- Be prepared in case you get sick and need to stay home for a week or so; a supply of over-the-counter medicines, alcohol-based hand rubs, tissues and other related items might could be useful and help avoid the need to make trips out in public while you are sick and contagious

(12) What is the best way to keep from spreading the virus through coughing or sneezing?

If you are sick with flu-like illness, CDC recommends that you stay home for at least 24 hours after your fever is gone except to get medical care or for other necessities. (Your fever should be gone without the use of a fever-reducing medicine.) Keep away from others as much as possible. Cover your mouth and nose with a tissue when coughing or sneezing. Put your used tissue in the waste basket. Then, clean your hands, and do so every time you cough or sneeze.

(13) If I have a family member at home who is sick with novel H1N1 flu, should I go to work?

Employees who are well but who have an ill family member at home with novel H1N1 flu can go to work as usual. These employees should monitor their health every day, and take everyday precautions including washing their hands often with soap and water, especially after they cough or sneeze. Alcohol-based hand cleaners are also effective. If they become ill, they should notify their supervisor and stay home. Employees who have an underlying medical condition or who are pregnant should call their health care provider for advice, because they might need to receive influenza antiviral drugs to prevent illness..

(14) What is the best technique for washing my hands to avoid getting the flu?

Washing your hands often will help protect you from

germs. Wash with soap and water or clean with alcohol-based hand cleaner. CDC recommends that when you wash your hands — with soap and warm water — that you wash for 15 to 20 seconds. When soap and water are not available, alcohol-based disposable hand wipes or gel sanitizers may be used. You can find them in most supermarkets and drugstores. If using gel, rub your hands until the gel is dry. The gel doesn't need water to work; the alcohol in it kills the germs on your hands.

(15) What should I do if I get sick?

If you live in areas where people have been identified with novel H1N1 flu and become ill with influenza-like symptoms, including fever, body aches, runny or stuffy nose, sore throat, nausea, or vomiting or diarrhea, you should stay home and avoid contact with other people. CDC recommends that you stay home for at least 24 hours after your fever is gone except to get medical care or for other necessities. (Your fever should be gone without the use of a fever-reducing medicine.) Stay away from others as much as possible to keep from making others sick.Staying at home means that you should not leave your home except to seek medical care. This means avoiding normal activities, including work, school, travel, shopping, social events, and public gatherings.

If you have severe illness or you are at high risk for flu complications, contact your health care provider or seek medical care. Your health care provider will determine whether flu testing or treatment is needed.

If you become ill and experience any of the warning signs (listed in chapter 4) seek emergency medical care.

(16) Are there medicines to treat novel H1N1 infection?

Yes. CDC recommends the use of oseltamivir or zanamivir for the treatment and/or prevention of infection with novel H1N1 flu virus. Antiviral drugs are prescription medicines (pills, liquid or an inhaled powder) that fight against the flu by keeping flu viruses from reproducing in your body. If you get sick, antiviral drugs can make your illness milder and make you feel better faster. They may also prevent serious flu complications. During the current pandemic, the priority use for influenza antiviral drugs during is to treat severe influenza illness (for example hospitalized patients) and people who are sick who have a condition that places them at high risk for serious flu-related complications.

(17) What is CDC's recommendation regarding "swine flu parties"?

"Swine flu parties" are gatherings during which people have close contact with a person who has novel H1N1 flu in order to become infected with the virus. The intent of these parties is for a person to become infected with what for many people has been a mild disease, in the hope of having natural immunity novel H1N1 flu virus that might circulate later and cause more severe disease.

CDC does not recommend "swine flu parties" as a way to protect against novel H1N1 flu in the future. While the disease seen in the current novel H1N1 flu outbreak has been mild for many people, it has been severe and even fatal for others. There is no way to predict with certainty what the outcome will be for an individual or, equally important, for others to whom the intentionally infected person may spread the virus.

Resistance to Antivirals

(18) How did WHO, the European Commission, the ECDC (European Centre for Disease Prevention and Control) and the European Medicines Agency learn about oseltamivir resistance in influenza viruses?

On 25 January 2008, the Norwegian authorities officially notified their EU partners and WHO, via the International Health Regulations (IHR) mechanism and the European Early Warning and Response System (EWRS) about a high rate of resistance to an antiviral drug, oseltamivir (Tamiflu©) in seasonal influenza A(H1N1) viruses. Of 16 virus isolates tested, 12 (75%) were resistant to oseltamivir. All the viruses were collected from patients earlier in the influenza season in November and December 2007 in Norway. Testing had been undertaken by National Institute of Public Health, the European Surveillance Network for Vigilance Against Viral Resistance (VIRGIL), the WHO Collaborating Center (CC) at the MRC National Institute for Medical Research in London and the European Influenza Surveillance Scheme (EISS).

(19) Has oseltamivir resistance been found in other countries this influenza season?

Yes, oseltamivir resistant H1N1 viruses have been identified in other countries this season. Testing by the VIRGIL through the EISS Network and ECDC, the WHO London CC, and National Influenza Centers (NICs) has found widely varying prevalences (0 to >60%) of H1N1 resistance among European countries (EU, EEA, EFTA countries), with Norway and France showing the highest levels to date.

WHO has sought further information from participants in its Global Influenza Surveillance Network (GISN) to assess the extent of circulation of oseltamivir-resistant viruses globally. None of the H1N1 isolates tested by the WHO CC in Tokyo or by China's Special Administrative Area of Hong Kong NIC were oseltamivir resistant last season (2006-7) or during the early part of the current season. The WHO CC at the Centers for Disease Control and Prevention in the United States has reported an 8% prevalence of resistance in H1N1 samples tested to date, and a similar prevalence of resistance has been detected in Canada. No resistance has been reported from Korea or New Zealand to date; two resistant variants detected in Australia were considered to be due to imported infections in travelers. However, resistance has been detected in some initially unaffected areas like Hong Kong among H1N1 isolates collected subsequently this season.

The available data indicate that oseltamivir resistance in H1N1 viruses is geographically variable both within Europe and globally. However, the distribution globally is not yet fully characterized and will likely change with time.

(20) Have other types of influenza viruses tested resistant to oseltamivir?

The elevated resistance to oseltamivir appears currently limited to seasonal H1N1 viruses and does not involve circulating H3N2 or influenza B viruses. All of the resistant H1N1 viruses in Europe have a specific resistance mutation in the viral neuraminidase (i.e., a histidine to tyrosine substitution at amino acid 274). Influenza H1N1 has been the predominant influenza A virus circulating (with a smaller contribution of influenza B viruses) in many countries in Europe and other parts of the northern hemisphere this season, but influenza A H3N2 or a mixture of A and B viruses have circulated in other countries. Furthermore, patterns may change as the season progresses.

(21) Is this a new problem?

Yes, the elevated prevalence of oseltamivir resistance in circulating H1N1 viruses in multiple countries is new. Resistance to oseltamivir in influenza viruses circulating in the community has been found before but at much lower levels. Past surveillance studies have found rates typically ranging from 0% to <0.5%. The highest rate of oseltamivir resistance that had been reported previously for surveillance of community isolates was in Japan during 2005-06 when 2.2 % of 178 H1N1 isolates were found to be resistant. During the last winter season (2006-7), no resistant H1N1 variants were detected in isolates from Japan or Europe, and less than 1% of U.S. H1N1 isolates showed oseltamivir resistance.

However, oseltamivir resistance is well-documented to emerge in persons being treated with the drug. In clinical studies, H1N1 viruses with this particular mutation have been detected in up to 16% of H1N1-infected children treated with oseltamivir. Typically, the resistant strains have emerged 3 to 6 days after treatment was begun but were not detected a few days later. However, past studies found little evidence of spread of resistant H1N1 virus to contacts or circulation within the community. The oseltamivir-resistant H1N1 viruses observed this year are different in that they are able to transmit from person to person.

(22) **Did resistance develop because patients in Norway and other countries were taking oseltamivir?**

None of the patients in Norway or elsewhere in Europe had been reported either to have taken oseltamivir beforehand or have been exposed to people who had taken oseltamivir. The lack of drug treatment is not unexpected since oseltamivir is not often prescribed by doctors in most European countries.

(23) **Is there an explanation for the high frequency of oseltamivir resistance?**

The frequency of oseltamivir resistance in H1N1 viruses in the current influenza season is unexpected and the reason why a high percentage of these viruses are resistant is currently unknown. Available information does not indicate selective drug pressure is driving the development of resistance since few of the patients are known to have taken oseltamivir. Influenza viruses are continuously changing and it is possible that a resistant strain has emerged spontaneously or has continued to spread in the community after being selected initially in someone treated with oseltamivir. Further detailed laboratory characterization of circulating H1N1 viruses and epidemiological information on patients will be needed to help answer this question.

(24) **Did the patients with resistant viruses have any links to one another?**

No. Preliminary investigations so far suggest that most of the persons with resistant viruses were not in contact or linked to each other or limited to a particular geographic location in a country. Not surprisingly, several household contacts affected by resistant H1N1 virus have been recognized. In general, patients in Norway or most other affected countries were not known to have traveled to other countries before becoming ill. These findings are consistent with this virus strain circulating at community level in some European and other countries.

(25) What sort of illness has been associated with the resistant viruses?

Information is limited at present, but there is no evidence that the resistant viruses are causing more or less severe illness than other influenza viruses. The Norwegian patients appear to have had typical influenza illness. Three of them were hospitalized and later discharged. Oseltamivir-resistant H1N1 viruses, similar to other seasonal influenza viruses, can cause severe disease and fatalities among vulnerable people such as infants and the elderly. However, influenza seasons in which H1N1 viruses predominate typically are associated with less severe illness and lower mortality overall than seasons in which H3N2 viruses are predominant.

(26) How easily are oseltamivir resistant viruses transmitted between people?

The available evidence indicates that these oseltamivir-resistant H1N1 viruses are transmissible from one person to another, but there is no evidence that the resistant H1N1 viruses are more transmissible between people than susceptible ones. Past studies in Japan suggested that low-level community transmission may occur with H1N1 viruses possessing the same resistance mutation that has been found in these recent cases. H1N1 viruses with this mutation are transmissible between laboratory animals.

(27) How does resistance affect oseltamivir's activity against the influenza virus?

Oseltamivir is an antiviral drug that blocks influenza viruses from spreading in the respiratory tract. The current resistant H1N1 viruses have been found to contain a specific mutation that makes them highly resistant to oseltamivir. This means that oseltamivir would most likely be ineffective for treating or preventing infections caused by these resistant H1N1 strains, although the drug will be effective against other influenza virus infections.

(28) Are there other drugs that can be used to treat oseltamivir resistant H1N1 virus infection?

To date all the oseltamivir-resistant H1N1 isolates this season have been fully susceptible to the other available antiviral drugs, zanamivir and the adamantanes (amantadine and rimantadine). These would be alternative drugs for prevention or treatment of oseltamivir-resistant H1N1 infections.

However, almost all influenza H3N2 viruses and, in some parts of the world, many H1N1 viruses are now resistant to the amantidine drugs. Consequently, effective use of these drugs would depend on knowledge of local patterns of circulating strains and their antiviral susceptibilities.

(29) Is this season's influenza vaccine effective against oseltamivir resistant strains?

The oseltamivir resistance mutation does not affect the vaccine's effectiveness, and there are no differences in antigenic properties between resistant and susceptible H1N1 viruses. Antiviral susceptibility and influenza vaccine effectiveness are based on different mechanisms. So far this influenza season, A(H1N1) viruses are predominant in most parts of northern hemisphere, and the majority are antigenically similar to A/Solomon Islands/3/2006, a vaccine virus, although an increasing proportion of recent H1N1 isolates have been antigenically distinguishable from the vaccine strain. Immunization with this season's vaccine remains an effective means of prevention against illness due to influenza viruses and should be comparably protective against oseltamivir-resistant and -susceptible H1N1 viruses.

(30) Do the oseltamivir resistant viruses pose any risk to cause a pandemic?

No, human seasonal H1N1 viruses, including those with a resistance mutation, do not have the potential to cause a pandemic. The current type of human H1N1 viruses have been circulating widely in the population for many years.

(31) **What potential implications could the findings of oseltamivir resistance among seasonal viruses have for the treatment of H5N1 cases?**

Oseltamivir resistance due to the same mutation has been reported in three patients with H5N1 infection who were treated with oseltamivir. There are no reports of persons acquiring H5N1 infection from a patient with an oseltamivir resistant H5N1 virus.

(32) **What implications does oseltamivir resistance in seasonal H1N1 viruses have for the avian influenza H5N1?**

The implications are uncertain at this point. The neuraminidase protein in human H1N1 viruses is different from that in avian H5N1 viruses. Until we learn why the unexpected increase in oseltamivir resistance has occurred in H1N1 viruses, it is too early to know what, if any, potential there might be for a similar increase in resistance to occur in H5N1 viruses. Furthermore, H5N1 viruses have not shown the ability to spread efficiently from person-to-person. WHO has not changed any of its recommendations regarding H5N1 treatment and preparations. A resistant human H1N1 virus could theoretically give its neuraminidase gene to an oseltamivir susceptible avian H5N1 virus if both viruses were to infect the same host. This is one way in which a resistant H5N1 could develop. However, none of the H5N1 viruses recovered from people have shown any evidence of such gene swapping to date. H5N1 viruses made from combinations of human and avian virus genes do not transmit or transmit very poorly in laboratory studies. Furthermore, H5N1 viruses have not shown the ability to spread efficiently from person-to-person.

(33) **What is being done about the situation?**

WHO, the European Commission and ECDC and other organizations worldwide are working together to gather additional information on antiviral resistance in H1N1 viruses. The Collaborating Centers in the WHO's Global Influenza Surveillance Network (GISN) and the VIRGIL

Network and the European Influenza Surveillance Scheme perform testing and share the results of antiviral susceptibility data on seasonal human viruses and H5N1 isolates. The WHO is also consulting with a variety of experts to assess the public health implications of these findings and the possible need for additional guidance.

(34) **What is going to happen? Is the oseltamivir resistant strain of H1N1 likely to become the predominant strain of H1N1 worldwide this influenza season?**

It is simply too early to know. Information to date indicates that the resistant virus is transmissible from person-to-person and that these viruses continue to circulate in some countries. However, the prevalence of resistant viruses varies widely in European and other countries. They are predominant only in Norway at present. Thus, it is possible that the resistant strain will not become more common in other countries this season or continue to circulate in future seasons. Careful monitoring will be required throughout the rest of the season to follow the situation globally.

(35) **How can I protect myself and my family from seasonal influenza?**

Seasonal influenza vaccination is the primary means of influenza prevention.

Following national guidance, people in high-risk groups for influenza complications (i.e. older persons, those with chronic conditions, etc) should be vaccinated against influenza, if they have not already done so.

- Seasonal vaccines are effective for those who wish to reduce their risk of influenza and some countries advise use in travellers to influenza-affected countries.

People can also take steps to reduce the spread of influenza:

- Where possible, people infected with influenza should avoid close contact with others.
- Basic hygiene measures, particularly covering coughs and sneezes and hand-washing, are likely effective in reducing the spread of influenza.

Antiviral drugs that are active against seasonal influenza viruses, including the resistant H1N1 virus, are available in many countries.

(36) What are the implications of this development for antiviral stockpiles?

The current H1N1 viruses are not a threat to cause a pandemic, and the cause and timing of the next influenza pandemic cannot be accurately predicted. Existing neuraminidase inhibitors, including oseltamivir, are useful against a range of influenza viruses, and oseltamivir resistance has been very uncommon in H5N1 viruses to date. The WHO and its partners will continue to carefully monitor antiviral susceptibility patterns in seasonal and animal influenza viruses. WHO is not making changes to its general advice on antiviral stockpiling for the time being.

Contamination and Cleaning

(37) How long can influenza virus remain viable on objects (such as books and doorknobs)?

Studies have shown that influenza virus can survive on environmental surfaces and can infect a person for 2 to 8 hours after being deposited on the surface.

(38) What kills influenza virus?

Influenza virus is destroyed by heat (167-212°F [75-100°C]). In addition, several chemical germicides, including chlorine, hydrogen peroxide, detergents (soap), iodophors (iodine-based antiseptics), and alcohols are effective against human influenza viruses if used in proper concentration for a sufficient length of time. For example, wipes or gels with alcohol in them can be used to clean hands. The gels should be rubbed into hands until they are dry.

(39) What if soap and water are not available and alcohol-based products are not allowed in my facility?

Though the scientific evidence is not as extensive as that on hand washing and alcohol-based sanitizers, other hand sanitizers that do not contain alcohol may be useful for killing flu germs on hands.

(40) What surfaces are most likely to be sources of contamination?

Germs can be spread when a person touches something that is contaminated with germs and then touches his or her eyes, nose, or mouth. Droplets from a cough or sneeze of an infected person move through the air. Germs can be spread when a person touches respiratory droplets from another person on a surface like a desk, for example, and then touches their own eyes, mouth or nose before washing their hands.

(41) How should waste disposal be handled to prevent the spread of influenza virus?

To prevent the spread of influenza virus, it is recommended that tissues and other disposable items used by an infected person be thrown in the trash. Additionally, persons should wash their hands with soap and water after touching used tissues and similar waste.

(42) What household cleaning should be done to prevent the spread of influenza virus?

To prevent the spread of influenza virus it is important to keep surfaces (especially bedside tables, surfaces in the bathroom, kitchen counters and toys for children) clean by wiping them down with a household disinfectant according to directions on the product label.

(43) How should linens, eating utensils and dishes of persons infected with influenza virus be handled?

Linens, eating utensils, and dishes belonging to those who are sick do not need to be cleaned separately, but importantly these items should not be shared without washing thoroughly first.

Linens (such as bed sheets and towels) should be washed by using household laundry soap and tumbled dry on a hot setting. Individuals should avoid "hugging" laundry prior to washing it to prevent contaminating themselves. Individuals should wash their hands with soap and water or alcohol-based hand rub immediately after handling dirty laundry.

Eating utensils should be washed either in a dishwasher or by hand with water and soap.

Transmission Routes

(44) Can I get infected with novel H1N1 virus from eating or preparing pork?

No. Novel H1N1 viruses are not spread by food. You cannot get infected with novel HIN1 virus from eating pork or pork products. Eating properly handled and cooked pork products is safe.

(45) Is there a risk from drinking water?

Tap water that has been treated by conventional disinfection processes does not likely pose a risk for transmission of influenza viruses. Current drinking water treatment regulations provide a high degree of protection from viruses. No research has been completed on the susceptibility of novel H1N1 flu virus to conventional drinking water treatment processes. However, recent studies have demonstrated that free chlorine levels typically used in drinking water treatment are adequate to inactivate highly pathogenic H5N1 avian influenza. It is likely that other influenza viruses such as novel H1N1 would also be similarly inactivated by chlorination. To date, there have been no documented human cases of influenza caused by exposure to influenza-contaminated drinking water.

(46) What surfaces are most likely to be sources of contamination?

Germs can be spread when a person touches something that is contaminated with germs and then touches his or her eyes, nose, or mouth. Droplets from a cough or sneeze of an infected person move through the air. Germs can be spread when a person touches respiratory droplets from another person on a surface like a desk, for example, and then touches their own eyes, mouth or nose before washing their hands.

(47) Can novel H1N1 flu virus be spread through water in swimming pools, spas, water parks, interactive fountains, and other treated recreational water venues?

Influenza viruses infect the human upper respiratory tract. There has never been a documented case of influenza virus infection associated with water exposure. Recreational water that has been treated at CDC recommended disinfectant levels does not likely pose a risk for transmission of influenza viruses. No research has been completed on the susceptibility of novel H1N1 influenza virus to chlorine and other disinfectants used in swimming pools, spas, water parks, interactive fountains, and other treated recreational venues.

However, recent studies have demonstrated that free chlorine levels recommended by CDC (1–3 parts per million [ppm or mg/L] for pools and 2–5 ppm for spas) are adequate to disinfect avian influenza A (H5N1) virus. It is likely that other influenza viruses such as novel H1N1 virus would also be similarly disinfected by chlorine.

(48) Can novel H1N1 influenza virus be spread at recreational water venues outside of the water?

Yes, recreational water venues are no different than any other group setting. The spread of this novel H1N1 flu is thought to be happening in the same way that seasonal flu spreads. Flu viruses are spread mainly from person to person through coughing or sneezing of people with influenza. Sometimes people may become infected by touching something with flu viruses on it and then touching their mouth or nose.

Surveillance

(49) Why did CDC stop reporting individual confirmed and probable novel H1N1 flu cases?

The case counts of novel H1N1 flu that were reported and updated weekly on the CDC website were based on reports of laboratory confirmed cases of influenza submitted by states. However, the number of cases of novel H1N1 flu infection continues to increase and most cases, particularly those that do not require hospitalization or those who do not seek medical care, are not tested. Therefore, the number of reported cases that are lab confirmed is a gross underestimation of the total number of illnesses.

Thus, on July 24, 2009 CDC transitioned from reporting probable and confirmed case counts to only reporting regional disease activity levels using its seasonal surveillance systems to track the progress of the novel H1N1 flu outbreak. This form of reporting disease activity levels is the method CDC uses to report on routine seasonal flu activity, which does not count individual cases, but instead monitors activity levels and virus characteristics through nine nationwide surveillance systems.

(50) Do you expect the virus to surge in the Fall? And if that's so, do you expect to it be worse than it has been?

We do expect seasonal influenza to return next fall or winter. Every year we see many strains of influenza circulate and the timing of the beginning of illness can vary from early to late fall to winter, depending on the part of the country. So that is a given. We are certain we will continue to have a seasonal problem with influenza. It is very possible that this virus will continue to circulate and cause much more illness again next fall or winter. Whether it will cause more illness than it has been causing recently, whether it will dominate among the seasonal flu viruses or whether it will really disappear is not predictable right now.

Other

(51) What is the difference between a vaccine and an antiviral?

Vaccines are usually given to prevent infections. Influenza vaccines are made from either pieces of the killed influenza virus or weakened versions of the live virus that will not lead to disease. When vaccinated, the body's immune system makes antibodies which will fight off infection if exposure to the virus occurs.

Antivirals are drugs that can treat people who have already been infected by a virus. They also can be used to prevent infection when given before or shortly after exposure and before illness occurs. A key difference between a vaccine and antiviral drug is that the antiviral drug will prevent infection only when administered within a certain time frame before or after exposure and is effective during the time that the drug is being taken while a vaccine can be given long before exposure to the virus and can provide protection over a long period of time.

(52) Is the swine flu virus mutating?

It is already a mutated form of the influenza virus. Influenza viruses are prone to mutate very rapidly, which is why even vaccination is not useful after a while, as the vaccination cannot protect against a new strain. There is fear that the virus could reassort with the seasonal flu viruses in the Southern hemisphere, where there is flu season going on. This could potentially make the virus even more deadly.

(53) Has the media exaggerated on the severity of the disease

The disease is actually like any other flu, except that it can be more dangerous in certain 'risk groups' that have been mentioned before. What the media has done, however, especially in India, is to report every single case, and that too standing outside hospitals with masks on. Such visuals have created a great deal of panic among people; making them all rush to hospitals to get themselves tested, consequently adding to the workload of hospital staffs. This also means that they are using up testing kits unnecessarily, which could potentially lead to their shortage.

APPENDIX

(A) SAFETY OF PANDEMIC VACCINES

Pandemic (H1N1) 2009 Briefing Note

The WHO is aware of some media reports that have expressed concern about the safety of vaccines for pandemic influenza. The public needs to be reassured that regulatory procedures in place for the licensing of pandemic vaccines, including procedures for expediting regulatory approval, are rigorous and do not compromise safety or quality controls.

Vaccines are among the most important medical interventions for reducing illness and deaths during a pandemic. However, to have the greatest impact, pandemic vaccines need to be available quickly and in large quantities.

During the 1957 and 1968 pandemics, vaccines arrived too late to be used as an effective mitigation tool during the more severe phases of the pandemics. Influenza vaccines had not yet been developed when the 1918 pandemic swept around the world, eventually killing an estimated 50 million people.

In 2007, as part of preparedness for an influenza pandemic, the WHO worked together with health officials, regulatory authorities, and vaccine manufacturers to explore a broad range of issues surrounding the regulatory approval of pandemic vaccines.

Ways were sought to shorten the time between the emergence of a pandemic virus and the availability of safe and effective vaccines. Different regulatory pathways were assessed and precautions needed to ensure quality, safety, and effectiveness were set out in detail.

Fast-Track Procedures for Approval

Regulatory authorities have shown great flexibility in developing procedures for fast tracking the approval and licensing of pandemic vaccines.

In some cases, pandemic vaccines are not regarded by regulatory authorities as entirely "new" vaccines, as they build on the technology used to produce vaccines for seasonal influenza, established procedures for testing and regulatory control, and an extensive body of safety data.

In such cases, approval procedures are similar to those applied to "strain changes" made each year when seasonal vaccines are modified to match circulating viruses in the Northern and Southern Hemispheres.

Specific regulatory procedures have been devised to expedite the approval of pandemic vaccines. In the USA, for example, fewer data are required when the manufacturer already has a licensed influenza vaccine and intends to use the same manufacturing process for its pandemic vaccine.

In the European Union, the European Medicines Agency uses a rolling review procedure whereby manufacturers can submit sets of data for regulatory review as they become available, without having to wait until all data can be submitted together in a single formal application.

Also in Europe, some manufacturers have conducted advance studies using a so-called "mock-up" vaccine. Mock-up vaccines contain an active ingredient for an influenza virus that has not circulated recently in human populations and thus mimics the novelty of a pandemic virus. Such advance studies can greatly expedite regulatory approval.

Special Safety Concerns

Influenza vaccines have been used for more than 60 years and have an established record of safety in all age groups. While some serious adverse events have been reported, these have been rare.

Nonetheless, special safety issues will inevitably arise during a pandemic when vaccine is administered on a massive scale. For example, adverse events too rare to show up even in a large clinical trial may become apparent when very large numbers of people receive a pandemic vaccine.

Some adverse events will be coincidental – that is, associated in time with vaccine administration, yet not directly caused by the vaccine. Genuine adverse events directly caused by the vaccine may also occur, but cannot be predicted in advance. Given the safety record of seasonal vaccines, such events are expected to be rare.

Time constraints mean that clinical data at the time when pandemic vaccines are first administered will inevitably be limited. Further testing of safety and effectiveness will need to take place after administration of the vaccine has begun.

For these reasons, WHO advises all countries administering pandemic vaccines to conduct intensive monitoring for safety and efficacy, and many countries have plans in place for doing so. On the positive side, mass vaccination campaigns can generate significant safety data within a few weeks.

International sharing of data from such post-marketing surveillance will be vital in guiding risk-benefit assessments and determining whether changes in vaccination policies are needed. WHO has developed standardized protocols for data collection and reporting in real-time, and will communicate findings to the international community via its web site.

(B) DETAILED TABLE OF H1N1 CASES

Confirmed Swine Flu Cases to Date

By date	By cont.	Country or territory	First case	April	May	June	July	August	Latest (5 Aug.)
0	0	World	2009-04-24	25	367	17398	77201	188333	199082
0	0	Days to double (approx)			2	15	15	28	29
0	0	Countries and territories		2	13	63	121	168	170
1	1.01	Mexico	2009-04-24	18	156	5029	8680	16442	17416
2	1.02	United States of America	2009-04-24	7	141	8975	27717	43771	43771
3	1.03	Canada	2009-04-27		34	1336	7983	10449	10449
16	1.04	Costa Rica	2009-05-02			37	279	668	755
19	1.05	El Salvador	2009-05-04			27	226	556	556
22	1.06	Guatemala	2009-05-06			12	254	558	558
27	1.07	Panama	2009-05-09			107	417	588	600
33	1.08	Cuba	2009-05-13			4	46	234	234
46	1.09	Honduras	2009-05-25			2	118	169	190
52	1.1	Dominican Republic	2009-05-29			2	108	154	154
59	1.11	Bahamas	2009-06-01			1	6	29	29
57	1.12	Jamaica	2009-06-01			2	32	62	62
67	1.13	Nicaragua	2009-06-03				293	432	472

(Contd.)

By date	By cont.	Country or territory	First case	April	May	June	July	August	Latest (5 Aug.)
68	1.14	Barbados	2009-06-05				10	23	31
72	1.15	Cayman Islands	2009-06-08				13	60	60
73	1.16	Dominica	2009-06-08				1	1	1
71	1.17	Trinidad and Tobago	2009-06-08				53	97	97
80	1.18	Bermuda	2009-06-17				1	4	4
81	1.19	British Virgin Islands	2009-06-17				1	5	5
83	1.2	Martinique	2009-06-17				2	3	3
84	1.21	Netherlands Antilles	2009-06-17				14	19	19
101	1.22	Antigua and Barbuda	2009-06-24				2	3	3
119	1.23	Saint Lucia	2009-07-01				1	3	3
122	1.24	Aruba	2009-06-03					13	13
127	1.25	Puerto Rico	2009-07-06					18	18
128	1.26	Guadeloupe	2009-07-06					2	2
131	1.27	Saint Martin	2009-07-06					1	1
132	1.28	US Virgin Islands	2009-07-06					1	1
143	1.29	St Vincent & the Grenadines	2009-07-10					1	1
147	1.30	Belize	2009-07-16					23	23
148	1.31	Haiti	2009-07-16					3	5
149	1.32	St Kitts & Nevis	2009-07-16					3	3
160	1.33	Grenada	2009-06-29					1	1
167	1.34	Turks & Caicos Is	2009-08-03					12	12
170	1.35	Anguilla	2009-08-05						1

4	2.01	Spain	2009-04-27	13	178	717	1538	1538
7	2.02	United Kingdom	2009-04-28	8	229	6538	11912	11912
9	2.03	Austria	2009-04-29	1	1	15	153	178
8	2.04	Germany	2009-04-29	4	28	417	6800	7963
10	2.05	Netherlands	2009-04-30	1	3	128	517	517
11	2.06	Switzerland	2009-04-30	1	8	56	484	535
13	2.07	Denmark	2009-05-01	1	1	55	254	280
14	2.08	France	2009-05-02		24	277	719	556
17	2.09	Ireland	2009-04-30		4	41	276	276
18	2.1	Italy	2009-05-03		29	123	975	975
21	2.11	Portugal	2009-05-04		1	17	342	354
23	2.12	Sweden	2009-05-06		4	69	526	551
24	2.13	Poland	2009-05-07		4	15	93	101
30	2.14	Norway	2009-05-11		4	32	471	607
31	2.15	Finland	2009-05-13		3	26	189	189
34	2.16	Belgium	2009-05-15		12	47	126	126
41	2.17	Greece	2009-05-20		4	92	730	730
43	2.18	Russia	2009-05-23		3	3	41	55
47	2.19	Iceland	2009-05-25		1	4	51	54
50	2.2	Romania	2009-05-29		3	28	178	194
53	2.21	Czech Republic	2009-05-29		1	9	116	135
54	2.22	Slovakia	2009-05-29		2	13	58	73
60	2.23	Cyprus	2009-06-01		1	48	297	297

(*Contd.*)

By date	By cont.	Country or territory	First case	April	May	June	July	August	Latest (5 Aug.)
61	2.24	Estonia	2009-06-01			1	13	42	44
62	2.25	Hungary	2009-06-01			1	10	99	102
65	2.26	Bulgaria	2009-06-03				67	36	36
69	2.27	Luxembourg	2009-06-05				4	61	61
75	2.28	Ukraine	2009-06-10				1	1	1
87	2.29	Isle of Man	2009-06-17				1	11	11
88	2.3	Jersey	2009-06-17				8	37	37
95	2.31	Slovenia	2009-06-22				4	136	150
105	2.32	Latvia	2009-06-24				1	19	19
106	2.33	Montenegro	2009-06-24				4	18	18
109	2.34	Serbia	2009-06-26				12	115	120
111	2.35	Guernsey	2009-06-26				5	18	18
115	2.36	Lithuania	2009-06-29				1	22	24
116	2.37	Monaco	2009-06-29					1	1
123	2.38	Malta	2009-06-03					157	168
124	2.39	Bosnia and Herzegovina	2009-06-03					2	10
129	2.40	Macedonia	2009-07-06					21	27
133	2.41	Croatia	2009-07-06					55	61
152	2.42	Georgia	2009-07-20					6	12
154	2.43	Albania	2009-07-22					3	13
161	2.44	Andorra	2009-06-29					1	1
162	2.45	Kosovo	2009-06-29					1	1

163	2.46	Azerbaijan	2009-07-31				2	2
164	2.47	Moldova	2009-07-31				1	2
166	2.48	Cyprus UK bases	2009-08-03				30	30
6	3.01	Israel	2009-04-28	2	19	506	1719	1719
12	3.02	China	2009-05-01	1	52	1518	6628	7126
15	3.03	Korea, Republic of	2009-05-02		33	202	1466	1550
26	3.04	Japan	2009-05-09		370	1266	5022	5022
32	3.05	Thailand	2009-05-13		2	1414	8879	10043
38	3.06	India	2009-05-17		1	104	551	574
37	3.07	Malaysia	2009-05-17		2	112	1446	1476
39	3.08	Turkey	2009-05-17		4	32	199	199
42	3.09	Philippines	2009-05-22		16	861	3207	3207
44	3.1	Taiwan	2009-05-23		12	61	1280	1280
45	3.11	Kuwait	2009-05-25		18	34	203	294
48	3.12	Bahrain	2009-05-27		1	15	123	130
49	3.13	Singapore	2009-05-27		5	701	1217	1217
63	3.14	Viet Nam	2009-06-01		1	123	971	995
66	3.15	Lebanon	2009-06-03			39	210	210
70	3.16	Saudi Arabia	2009-06-05			81	595	595
74	3.17	United Arab Emirates	2009-06-08			8	110	125
76	3.18	West Bank and Gaza Strip	2009-06-15			13	104	81
78	3.19	Qatar	2009-06-17			10	43	43
79	3.2	Jordan	2009-06-17			20	79	79

(Contd.)

By date	By cont.	Country or territory	First case	April	May	June	July	August	Latest (5 Aug.)
86	3.21	Sri Lanka	2009-06-17				15	55	60
89	3.22	Yemen	2009-06-17				7	11	11
91	3.23	Oman	2009-06-19				3	123	125
92	3.24	Laos	2009-06-19				3	51	156
93	3.25	Papua New Guinea	2009-06-19				1	1	1
96	3.26	Bangladesh	2009-06-22				1	30	32
97	3.27	Brunei	2009-06-22				29	786	786
107	3.28	Cambodia	2009-06-24				6	17	21
110	3.29	Indonesia	2009-06-26				8	561	662
112	3.3	Iran	2009-06-26				1	105	124
113	3.31	Iraq	2009-06-29				1	58	58
114	3.32	Nepal	2009-06-29				11	17	17
120	3.33	Myanmar	2009-07-01				1	10	13
134	3.34	Syria	2009-07-06					5	9
137	3.35	Afghanistan	2009-07-08					32	32
156	3.36	Bhutan	2009-06-27					2	3
157	3.37	Maldives	2009-06-27					1	1
158	3.38	Kazakhstan	2009-06-29					14	15
168	3.39	Pakistan	2009-08-03					1	1
5	4.01	New Zealand	2009-04-28		4	9	711	2855	2893
29	4.02	Australia	2009-05-09			297	4090	22109	24114
82	4.03	French Polynesia	2009-06-17				2	16	16

85	4.04	Samoa	2009-06-17				1	37	37
98	4.05	Fiji	2009-06-22				2	97	97
108	4.06	Vanuatu	2009-06-24				2	3	3
118	4.07	New Caledonia	2009-07-01				6	112	112
125	4.08	Palau	2009-06-03					1	1
135	4.09	Cook Islands	2009-07-06					1	1
142	4.10	Guam	2009-07-10					1	1
144	4.11	Tonga	2009-07-15					9	9
153	4.12	Solomon Islands	2009-07-22					2	3
155	4.13	Micronesia	2009-07-22					1	1
20	5.01	Colombia	2009-05-04			20	93	270	275
25	5.02	Brazil	2009-05-08			20	680	1958	2959
28	5.03	Argentina	2009-05-09			100	1587	3056	4895
35	5.04	Ecuador	2009-05-16			39	163	696	696
36	5.05	Peru	2009-05-16			36	538	4104	4889
40	5.06	Chile	2009-05-18			250	6211	11860	11860
51	5.07	Uruguay	2009-05-29			11	195	550	550
55	5.08	Paraguay	2009-06-01			5	205	223	223
56	5.09	Bolivia	2009-06-01			3	96	946	969
58	5.1	Venezuela	2009-06-01			2	193	454	476
90	5.11	Suriname	2009-06-19				11	14	14
130	5.12	Guyana	2009-07-06					5	6

(Contd.)

By date	By cont.	Country or territory	First case	April	May	June	July	August	Latest (5 Aug.)
146	5.13	French Guiana	2009-07-13					9	9
169	5.14	Falkland Is	2009-08-05						5
66	6.01	Egypt	2009-06-03				39	283	289
77	6.02	Morocco	2009-06-15				17	66	71
94	6.03	South Africa	2009-06-19				1	480	700
99	6.04	Algeria	2009-06-22				2	16	16
100	6.05	Cape Verde	2009-06-24				3	6	6
102	6.06	Cote d'Ivoire	2009-06-24				2	2	2
103	6.07	Tunisia	2009-06-24				3	10	10
104	6.08	Ethiopia	2009-06-24				2	4	4
117	6.09	Mauritius	2009-07-01				7	2	2
121	6.1	Kenya	2009-07-01				1	26	26
126	6.11	Uganda	2009-06-03					9	9
136	6.12	Libya	2009-07-06					9	9
138	6.13	Réunion	2009-07-08					26	26
139	6.14	Seychelles	2009-07-08					3	3
140	6.15	Tanzania	2009-07-09					8	10
145	6.16	Botswana	2009-07-13					13	23
150	6.17	Sudan	2009-07-17					2	2
151	6.18	Namibia	2009-07-20					4	5
159	6.19	Swaziland	2009-06-29					2	2
165	6.20	Gabon	2009-07-31					1	1

(C) DETAILS OF DEATHS BY SWINE FLU

By date	By cont.	Country	First death	April	May	June	July	August	Latest (Aug. 5)
0	0	World	2009-04-27		10	115	332	1265	1444
0	0	Countries		0	2	4	17	45	48
1	1.01	Mexico	2009-04-27		9	97	116	146	146
2	1.02	USA	2009-04-30		1	15	127	353	353
3	1.03	Canada	2009-05-09			2	25	59	62
4	1.04	Costa Rica	2009-05-10			1	2	22	25
6	1.05	Dominican Republic	2009-06-08				2	5	5
8	1.06	Guatemala	2009-06-12				2	10	10
13	1.07	Honduras	2009-06-26				1	4	6
21	1.08	El Salvador	2009-07-08					9	12
22	1.09	Jamaica	2009-07-08					3	3
30	1.10	Panama	2009-07-22					2	2
37	1.11	Cayman Is.	2009-07-29					1	1
38	1.12	St Kitts and Nevis	2009-07-29					1	1
5	2.01	Chile	2009-06-05				12	87	96
7	2.02	Colombia	2009-06-11				2	17	17

(Contd.)

By date	By cont.	Country	First death	April	May	June	July	August	Latest (Aug. 5)
9	2.03	Argentina	2009-06-15				26	165	243
15	2.04	Brazil	2009-07-01				1	56	96
16	2.05	Uruguay	2009-07-01				1	22	22
19	2.06	Paraguay	2009-07-06					19	19
20	2.07	Peru	2009-07-08					30	33
24	2.08	Ecuador	2009-07-10					18	19
25	2.09	Bolivia	2009-07-19					9	11
27	2.10	Venezuela	2009-07-20					2	2
10	3.01	UK	2009-06-17				3	30	30
17	3.02	Spain	2009-07-01				1	7	8
33	3.03	Hungary	2009-07-24					1	1
40	3.04	Belgium	2009-07-31					1	1
43	3.05	France	2009-07-31					1	1
47	3.06	Netherlands	2009-08-05						1
11	4.01	Australia	2009-06-19				7	67	74
18	4.02	New Zealand	2009-07-06					14	14
31	4.03	Tonga	2009-07-22					1	1
12	5.01	Philippines	2009-06-24				1	8	8
14	5.02	Thailand	2009-07-01				3	65	81
23	5.03	Brunei	2009-07-08					1	1

26	5.04	China	2009-07-16	3	3
28	5.05	Singapore	2009-07-20	6	6
32	5.06	Laos	2009-07-22	1	1
34	5.07	Indonesia	2009-07-27	1	3
35	5.08	Malaysia	2009-07-29	7	11
36	5.09	Saudi Arabia	2009-07-29	4	6
39	5.10	Israel	2009-07-29	2	2
42	5.11	Taiwan	2009-07-31	1	1
45	[illegible]	Lebanon	2009-07-30	1	1
46	5.13	Qatar	2009-08-03	1	1
47	5.14	India	2009-08-12		13
48	5.15	Vietnam	2009-08-05		1
29	6.01	Egypt	2009-07-20	1	1
44	6.02	South Africa	2009-08-03	1	1

Glossary

Acute: Of abrupt onset, in reference to a disease. Acute often also connotes an illness that is of short duration, rapidly progressive, and in need of urgent care.

Airway: The path air follows to get into and out of the lungs. The mouth and nose are the normal entry and exit ports. Entering air then passes through the back of the throat (pharynx), continues through the voice box (larynx), down the trachea, and finally out the branching tubes known as bronchi.

Allergic Reaction: The hypersensitive response of the immune system of an allergic individual to a substance.

Antigenic Drift: A mechanism for variation by viruses that involves the accumulation of mutations within the antibody-binding sites so that the resulting viruses cannot be inhibited well by antibodies against previous strains making it easier for them to spread throughout a partially immune population. Antigenic drift occurs in both Influenza A and Influenza B viruses.

Antigenic Shift: A sudden shift in the antigenicity of a virus resulting from the recombination of the genomes of two viral strains. Antigenic shift is seen only with influenza A viruses. It results usually from the replacement of the hemagglutinin (the viral attachment protein that also mediates the entry of the virus into the cell) with a novel subtype that has not been present in human Influenza Viruses for a long time. The consequences of the introduction of a new hemagglutinin into human viruses is usually a pandemic, or a worldwide epidemic.

Antiviral: An agent that kills a virus or that suppresses its ability to replicate and, hence, inhibits its capability to multiply and reproduce.

Asymptomatic: Without symptoms. An asymptomatic infection is an infection with no symptoms.

B virus: An infectious agent commonly found among macaque monkeys, including rhesus macaques, pig-tailed macaques, and cynomolgus monkeys. Monkeys infected with this virus usually have no or mild symptoms. In humans, however, B virus infection can result in a fatal encephalomyelitis. B virus disease in humans is extremely rare, but often fatal — an estimated 80% of untreated patients die of complications associated with the infection.

Bacterial: Of or pertaining to bacteria. For example, a bacterial lung infection.

Carrier: A person apparently in good health harbouring a pathogenic microorganism.

CDC: The Centers for Disease Control and Prevention, the US agency charged with tracking and investigating public health trends. The stated mission of the CDC is "To promote health and quality of life by preventing and controlling disease, injury, and disability." The CDC is a part of the U.S. Public Health Services (PHS) under the Department of Health and Human Services (HHS).

Cell: The basic structural and functional unit in people and all living things. Each cell is a small container of chemicals and water wrapped in a membrane.

Centre for Disease Control and Prevention: The US agency charged with tracking and investigating public health trends. The stated mission of the Centers for Disease Control and Prevention, commonly called the CDC, is "To promote health and quality of life by preventing and controlling disease, injury, and disability."

Chemoprophylaxis: The use of a chemical agent to prevent the development of a disease.

Chills: feelings of coldness accompanied by shivering. Chills may develop after exposure to a cold environment or may accompany a fever.

Chronic: This important term in medicine comes from the Greek *chronos,* time and means lasting a long time.

Complication: In medicine, an additional problem that arises following a procedure, treatment or illness and is secondary to it. A complication complicates the situation.

Congestion: An abnormal or excessive accumulation of a body fluid. The term is used broadly in medicine. Examples include nasal congestion (excess mucus and secretions in the air passages of the nose) seen with a common cold and congestion of blood in the lower extremities seen with some types of heart failure.

Conjunctivitis: Inflammation of the conjunctiva, the membrane on the inner part of the eyelids and the membrane covering the white of the eye. The conjunctival membranes react to a wide range of bacteria, viruses, allergy-provoking agents, irritants and toxic agents. Viral and bacterial forms of conjunctivitis are common in childhood. Conjunctivitis is also called pinkeye and red eye.

Coronavirus: One of a group of RNA viruses, so named because they look like a corona or halo when viewed under the electron microscope. The corona or halo is due to an array of surface projections on the viral envelope.

Cough: A rapid expulsion of air from the lungs typically in order to clear the lung airways of fluids, mucus, or material. Also called *tussis.*

Cytokine: Chemicals which are used by immune cells to communicate with each other; when the cells have to respond to any foreign substance.

Diarrhoea: A familiar phenomenon with unusually frequent or unusually liquid bowel movements, excessive watery evacuations of fecal material. The opposite of constipation . The word "diarrhea" with its odd spelling is a near steal from the Greek "diarrhoia" meaning "a flowing through." Plato and Aristotle may have had diarrhoia while today we have diarrhea. There are myriad infectious and noninfectious causes of diarrhea.

Dyspnea: Difficult or labored breathing; shortness of breath.

Epidemic: The occurrence of more cases of a disease than would be expected in a community or region during a given time period. A sudden severe outbreak of a disease such as SARS. From the Greek "epi-", "upon" + "demos", "people or population" = "epidemos" = "upon the population." See also: Endemic; Pandemic.

Exacerbation: A worsening. In medicine, exacerbation may refer to an increase in the severity of a disease or its signs and symptoms. For example, exacerbation of asthma is one of the serious effects of air pollution..

Fatigue: A condition characterized by a lessened capacity for work and reduced efficiency of accomplishment, usually accompanied by a feeling of weariness and tiredness. Fatigue can be acute and come on suddenly or chronic and persist.

FDA: The Food and Drug Administration, an agency within the U.S. Public Health Service, which is a part of the Department of Health and Human Services.

Febrile: Feverish.

Fever : Although a fever technically is any body temperature above the normal of 98.6 degrees F. (37 degrees C.), in practice a person is usually not considered to have a significant fever until the temperature is above 100.4 degrees F (38 degrees C.)

Flu: Short for influenza. The flu is caused by viruses that infect the respiratory tract which are divided into three types, designated A, B, and C. Most people who get the flu recover completely in 1 to 2 weeks, but some people develop serious and potentially life-threatening medical complications, such as pneumonia. Much of the illness and death caused by influenza can be prevented by annual influenza vaccination.

Formalin: A 37% aqueous (water) solution of formaldehyde, a pungent gas, with the chemical formula HCHO, used as an antiseptic, disinfectant, and especially today as a fixative for histology (the study of tissues under the microscope).

Gastrointestinal: Adjective referring collectively to the stomach and small and large intestines.

Genetic: Having to do with genes and genetic information.

Genetic code: The instructions in a gene that tell the cell how to make a specific protein. A, T, G, and C are the "letters" of the DNA code. They stand for the chemicals adenine, thymine, guanine, and cytosine, respectively, which make up the nucleotide bases of DNA. Each gene's code combines the four chemicals in various ways to spell out 3-letter "words" that specify which amino acid is needed at every step in making a protein.

Genome: All of the genetic information, the entire genetic complement, all of the hereditary material possessed by an organism.

Headache: A pain in the head with the pain being above the eyes or the ears, behind the head (occipital), or in the back of the upper neck. Headache, like chest pain or backache, has many causes.

Hygiene: The science of preventive medicine and the preservation of health. From the name of Hygeia, the daughter of Asklepios, the Greek god of medicine (whose staff with entwined snake is the symbol of medicine). Asklepios (known to the Romans as Aesculapius) had a number of children including not only Hygeia but also Panaceia, the patroness of clinical medicine. Hygeia also followed her father into medicine. As the patroness of health, Hygeia was charged with providing a healthy environment to prevent illness. In Greek, "hygieia" means health.

Immune: Protected against infection. The Latin immunis means free, exempt.

Immune response: Any reaction by the immune system.

Infection: The growth of a parasitic organism within the body. (A parasitic organism is one that lives on or in another organism and draws its nourishment therefrom.) A person with an infection has another organism (a "germ") growing within him, drawing its nourishment from the person.

Influenza: The flu is caused by viruses that infect the respiratory tract which are divided into three types, designated A, B, and C. Most people who get the flu recover completely in 1 to 2 weeks, but some people develop serious and potentially life-threatening medical complications, such as pneumonia. Much of the illness and death caused by influenza can be prevented by annual influenza vaccination.

Laboratory: A place for doing tests and research procedures and preparing chemicals, etc. Although "laboratory" looks very like the Latin "laboratorium" (a place to labor, a work place), the word "laboratory" came from the Latin "elaborare" (to work out, as a problem, and with great pains), as evidenced by the Old English spelling "elaboratory" designating "a place where learned effort was applied to the solution of scientific problems."

Lungs: The lungs are a pair of breathing organs located with the chest which remove carbon dioxide from and bring oxygen to the blood. There is a right and left lung.

Mortality: A fatal outcome or, in one word, death. The word "mortality" is derived from "mortal" which came from the Latin "mors" (death). The opposite of mortality is, of course, immortality. Mortality is also quite distinct from morbidity (illness).

Mortality rate: A death rate. There are a number of different types of mortality rates as, for examples, the following:

- The *Foetal Mortality Rate*: The ratio of foetal deaths to the sum of the births (the live births + the foetal deaths) in that year.

- The *Infant Mortality Rate*: The number of children dying under a year of age divided by the number of live births that year.
- The *Maternal Mortality Rate*: The number of maternal deaths related to childbearing divided by the number of live births (or by the number of live births + foetal deaths) in that year.

Mouth: **1.** The upper opening of the digestive tract, beginning with the lips and containing the teeth, gums, and tongue. Foodstuffs are broken down mechanically in the mouth by chewing and saliva is added as a lubricant. Saliva contains amylase, an enzyme that digests starch. **2.** Any opening or aperture in the body. The mouth in both senses of the word is also called the *os*, the Latin word for an opening, or mouth.

Myalgia: Pain in a muscle; or pain in multiple muscles. Myalgia means muscle pain. There are many specific causes of various types of myalgia. Myalgia can be temporary or chronic. Myalgia can be a result of a mild conditions, such as a virus infection, or from a more serious illness. Examples include epidemic myalgia and polymyalgia rheumatica.

Nasal: Having to do with the nose. Nasal drops are intended for the nose, not (for example) the eyes. The word "nasal" came from the Latin "nasus" meaning the nose or snout.

Nausea: the urge to vomit. It can be brought by many causes including, systemic illnesses, such as influenza, medications, pain, and inner ear disease. When nausea and/or vomiting are persistent, or when they are accompanied by other severe symptoms such as abdominal pain, jaundice, fever, or bleeding, a physician should be consulted.

Neurological: Having to do with the nerves or the nervous system.

Nose: The external midline projection from the face.

Onset: In medicine, the first appearance of the signs or symptoms of an illness as, for example, the onset of rheumatoid arthritis . There is always an onset to a disease but never to the return to good health. The default setting is good health.

Pandemic: An epidemic (a sudden outbreak) that becomes very widespread and affects a whole region, a continent, or the world.

Pneumonia: Inflammation of one or both lungs with consolidation. Pneumonia is frequently but not always due to infection. The infection may be bacterial, viral, fungal or parasitic. Symptoms may include fever, chills, cough with sputum production, chest pain, and shortness of breath.

Pregnancy: The state of carrying a developing embryo or fetus within the female body. This condition can be indicated by positive results on an over-the-counter urine test, and confirmed through a blood test, ultrasound, detection of fetal heartbeat, or an X-ray. Pregnancy lasts for about nine months, measured from the date of the woman's last menstrual period (LMP). It is conventionally divided into three trimesters, each roughly three months long.

Prognosis: **1.** The expected course of a disease.

2. The patient's chance of recovery. The prognosis predicts the outcome of a disease and therefore the future for the patient.

Public Health: The approach to medicine that is concerned with the health of the community as a whole. Public health is community health. It has been said that: "Health care is vital to all of us some of the time, but public health is vital to all of us all of the time."

Quarantine: The period of isolation decreed to control the spread of infectious disease. Before the era of antibiotics, quarantine was one of the few available means for halting the spread of infectious diseases. It is still employed as needed. The list of quarantinable diseases in the US includes cholera, diphtheria, infectious tuberculosis, plague, smallpox, yellow fever, and viral hemorrhagic fevers (such as Marburg, Ebola and Congo-Crimean disease). In 2003, SARS (severe acute respiratory syndrome) was added as a quarantinable disease.

Resistance: Opposition to something, or the ability to withstand it. For example, some forms of staphylococcus are resistant to treatment with antibiotics.

Respiratory: Having to do with respiration, the exchange of oxygen and carbon dioxide. From the Latin re- (again) + spirare (to breathe) = to breathe again.

Respiratory failure: Inability of the lungs to perform their basic task of gas exchange, the transfer of oxygen from inhaled air into the blood and the transfer of carbon dioxide from the blood into exhaled air. The basis of respiratory failure may be failure of the exchange of oxygen and carbon dioxide within the tiny air sacs (alveoli) in the lungs; failure of the muscles required to expand the lungs; or failure of the brain centers controlling respiration.

Rhinorrhea: Medical term for a runny nose. From the Greek words "rhinos" meaning "of the nose" and "rhoia" meaning "a flowing."

RNA: Short for ribonucleic acid, a nucleic acid molecule similar to DNA but containing ribose rather than deoxyribose. RNA is formed upon a DNA template. There are several classes of RNA molecules.

SARS: Severe acute respiratory syndrome. A severe form of pneumonia which appeared in outbreaks in 2003.

Sneeze: **1.** As a verb, to suddenly expel air through the nose and mouth by an involuntary contraction of the muscles of expiration. **2.** As a noun, the act of sneezing.

Sore: **1.** (adjective) A popular term for painful. I have sore fingers from typing dictionary terms. She has a sore throat **2.** (noun) A nondescript term for nearly any lesion of the skin or mucous membranes. He has a number of sores in his mouth.

Sore Throat: Pain in the throat. Sore throat may be caused by many different causes, including inflammation of the larynx, pharynx, or tonsils.

Spanish Flu: A pandemic of influenza A (H1N1) in 1918-19 that caused the highest number of known flu deaths. More than 500,000 people died in the United States, and 20 million to

50 million people may have died worldwide. Many people died within the first few days after infection and others died of complications soon after. Nearly half of those who died were young, healthy adults. Also known as Spanish influenza.

Stage: As regards cancer, the extent of a cancer, especially whether the disease has spread from the original site to other parts of the body.

Strain: 1. An injury to a tendon or muscle resulting from overuse or trauma. 2. A hereditary tendency that originated from a common ancestor. 3. To exert maximum effort. 4. To filter.

Swine flu: A respiratory illness of pigs caused by infection with swine influenza A virus (SIV). While swine flu viruses normally do not infect humans, occasional infections of humans do occur. Many human cases of swine influenza A virus infection occur in individuals who have had a history of recent direct contact with pigs or close (within 6 feet) contact with pigs. Rare instances of human-to-human transmission have been documented. Swine flu infections have also occurred in individuals with no history of exposure to pigs. Symptoms typically range from a mild respiratory illness to flu-like symptoms with fever. Treatment involves the use of antiviral medications begun as soon as possible after the onset of symptoms. There is no human vaccine to protect against swine flu, although vaccines are available to be given to pigs to prevent swine flu.

Symptomatic: **1** With symptoms, as a symptomatic infection. **2** Characteristic, as behavior symptomatic of Huntington disease. **3** Directed at the symptoms, asymptomatic treatment.

Syndrome: A set of signs and symptoms that tend to occur together and which reflect the presence of a particular disease or an increased chance of developing a particular disease.

Teratogenic: Able to disturb the growth and development of an embryo or fetus.

Throat: The throat is the anterior (front) portion of the neck beginning at the back of the mouth, consisting anatomically of the pharynx and larynx . The throat contains the trachea and a portion of the esophagus.

Trimester: The nine months of pregnancy is traditionally divided into three trimesters: distinct periods of roughly three months in which different phases of fetal development take place.

Vaccination: Injection of a killed microbe in order to stimulate the immune system against the microbe, thereby preventing disease. Vaccinations, or immunizations, work by stimulating the immune system, the natural disease-fighting system of the body. The healthy immune system is able to recognize invading bacteria and viruses and produce substances (antibodies) to destroy or disable them. Immunizations prepare the immune system to ward off a disease. To immunize against viral diseases, the virus used in the vaccine has been weakened or killed. To only immunize against bacterial diseases, it is generally possible to use a small portion of the dead bacteria to stimulate the formation of antibodies against the whole bacteria. In addition to the initial immunization process, it has been found that the effectiveness of immunizations can be improved by periodic repeat injections or "boosters." Also see Vaccines (in the plural) and Vaccine of a specific type (such Vaccine, Polio).

Vaccines: Microbial preparations of killed or modified microorganisms that can stimulate an immune response in the body to prevent future infection with similar microorganisms. These preparations are usually delivered by injection.

Ventilation: The exchange of air between the lungs and the atmosphere so that oxygen can be exchanged for carbon dioxide in the alveoli (the tiny air sacs in the lungs).

Ventilator: A ventilator is a machine which mechanically assists patients in the exchange of oxygen and carbon dioxide (sometimes referred to as artificial respiration).

Viable: Capable of life. For example, a viable premature baby is one who is able to survive outside the womb.

Viral: Of or pertaining to a virus. For example, "My daughter has a viral rash."

Viral infection: Infection caused by the presence of a virus in the body. Depending on the virus and the person's state of health, various viruses can infect almost any type of body tissue, from the brain to the skin. Viral infections cannot be treated with antibiotics; in fact, in some cases the use of antibiotics makes the infection worse. The vast majority of human viral infections can be effectively fought by the body's own immune system, with a little help in the form of proper diet, hydration, and rest. As for the rest, treatment depends on the type and location of the virus, and may include anti-viral or other drugs.

Virus: A microorganism smaller than a bacteria, which cannot grow or reproduce apart from a living cell. A virus invades living cells and uses their chemical machinery to keep itself alive and to replicate itself. It may reproduce with fidelity or with errors (mutations)-this ability to mutate is responsible for the ability of some viruses to change slightly in each infected person, making treatment more difficult.

Viruses: Small living particles that can infect cells and change how the cells function. Infection with a virus can cause a person to develop symptoms. The disease and symptoms that are caused depend on the type of virus and the type of cells that are infected.

Voluntary: Done in accordance with the conscious will of the individual. The opposite of involuntary.

World Health Organization: An agency of the United Nations established in 1948 to further international cooperation in improving health conditions. Although the World Health Organization inherited specific tasks relating to epidemic control, quarantine measures, and drug standardization from the Health Organization of the League of Nations (that was set up in 1923) and from the International Office of Public

Health at Paris (established in 1909), the World Health Organization was given a broad mandate under its constitution to promote the attainment of "the highest possible level of health" by all people. WHO defines health positively as "a state of complete physical, mental, and social well-being and not merely the absence of disease or infirmity."

Important Acronyms

AIIMS	All India Institute of Medical Sciences
AIMC	Avian Influenza Monitoring Cell
APHO	Air Port Health Organization
BDO	Block Development Officer
BSL	Bio Safety Laboratory
CDC	Centre for Disease Control
CHC	Community Health Centre
CISF	Central Industrial Security Force
CMO	Chief Medical Officer (of the District)
CRB	Consciousness, Respiration and Blood Pressure
CRI	Central Research Institute, Kasuali
DDMA	District Disaster Management Authority
DGHS	Director General of Health Services
Dte GHS	Directorate General of Health Services
DHS	Director of Health Services (State)
DM	District Magistrate
ADM	Additional District Megistrate
EMR	Emergency Medical Relief Division
EOC	Emergency Operating Centre
ESF	Emergency Support Function (plan of MOHFW)
ESI	Employees State Insurance Corporation
JMG	Joint Monitoring Group.
I&B	Information and Broadcasting

ICMR	Indian Council of Medical Research
IDSP	Integrated Disease Surveillance Project
IEC	Information, Education, Communication
IHR	International Health Regulation
ILI	Influenza Like Illness
IMA	Indian Medical Association
IMTF	Inter Ministerial Task Force
MOHFW	Ministry of Health and Family Welfare
MHA	Ministry of Home Affairs
NCMC	National Crisis Management Committee
NCC	National Cadet Corps
NDMA	National Disaster Management Authority
NGO	Non Governmental Organization
NIC	National Influenza Centre
NICD	National Institute of Communicable Diseases
NICED	National Institute of Cholera and Enteric Diseases
NIV	National Institute of Virology
NRHM	National Rural Health Mission
NSS	National Social Service
PHC	Primary Health Centre
PPE	Personal Protective Equipment
PRI	Panchayati Raj Institutions
PWD	Public Work Department
RMRC	Regional Medical Research Centre
ROHFW	Regional Office of Health and Family Welfare
RRT	Rapid Response Team
SARI	Severe Acute Respiratory Disease.
SDMA	State Disaster Management Authority
SOP	Standard Operating Procedure
SP	Superintendent of Police
UN	United Nations
UNICEF	United Nations Children Fund
WHO	World Health Organization

Bibliography/Websites/Links

- Ananthanarayan and Panicker's: Textbook of Microbiology.
- Morgan: The Genetics Revolution.
- Friefelder: Molecular Biology.
- Everson: The Gene.
- European Centre for Disease Prevention and Control: Update: "ECDC Situation Report, 11 August 2009". 2009-08-12 17:00 UTC +2. Retrieved on 2009-08-12.
- "Pandemic (H1N1) 2009 - update 60". World Health Organization. 2009-07-31. Retrieved on 2009-08-05.
- Sum of state reported confirmed and suspected cases; See US Swine Flu outbreak table for more information.
- "Total U.S. Novel H1N1 Flu Hospitalizations and Deaths". CDC. 2009-08-07. Retrieved on 2009-08-08.
- "INFLUENZA PANDÉMICA (H1N1) 2009. REPÚBLICA ARGENTINA - SEMANA EPIDEMIOLÓGICA Nº 30". Ministerio de Salud. 2009-08-01. Retrieved on 2009-08-05.
- "Regional Update Pandemic (H1N1) 2009". PAHO. 2009-07-31. Retrieved on 2009-08-04.
- http://portal.saude.gov.br/portal/arquivos/pdf/informe_influenza_se30_03_08_2009.pdf.
- "Rio registra mais 2 mortes por gripe suína; total vai a 210". Terra. 2009-08-11. Retrieved on 2009-08-11.
- "En dos días, 311 nuevos casos de contagio por influenza". 2009-08-06. Retrieved on 2009-08-07.
- "Mexico confirms 42 deaths of A/H1N1 flu". 2009-05-07. Retrieved on 2009-05-29. "Cordova said [...] 77 [early deaths] did not have

usable samples, meaning that they would never be confirmed or ruled out.".

- "National H1N1 Influenza 09 Update 12 noon 11 August 2009". Department of Health and Ageing. Retrieved on 2009-08-11.
- "A/H1N1 flu situation on Chile". 2009-08-05. Retrieved on 2009-08-05.
- "Summary of Situation of Pandemic H1N1 2009 for week of 27 July - 2 August 2009". WHO SEARO. Retrieved on 2009-08-06.
- "Flu vaccine trial gets the go-ahead". Bangkok Post. 2009-08-11. Retrieved on 2009-08-11.
- "Thailand's death toll from flu A/H1N1 rises to 97". Xinhua. 2009-08-11. Retrieved on 2009-08-11.
- Sum of Canadian province-reported confirmed cases; See Canadian Swine Flu outbreak table for more information.
- "B.C.'s H1N1 death toll climbs to 4, pushing national swine flu toll to 65". AFP. 2009-08-11. Retrieved on 2009-08-11.
- "Fallecidos por gripe AH1N1 en el Perú se elevó a 40" (in Spanish). RPP.com. 2009-08-08. Retrieved on 2009-08-08.
- "Fallecidos por gripe AH1N1 en el Perú se elevó a 40" (in Spanish). RPP.com. 2009-08-08. Retrieved on 2009-08-08.
- "EuroFlu - Weekly Electronic Bulletin Week 31: 27/07/2009-02/08/2009". WHO Europe. 2009-08-07. Retrieved on 2009-08-07.
- North Ireland: L+ / * / low
  Scotland: W+ / ** / low
  Wales: W+ / * / mod
  Source: WHO update 60 / *EuroFlu week* 31.
- "HPA Weekly National Influenza Report". *Week* 32. UK HPA. 2009-08-06. Retrieved on 2009-08-06.
- http://www.mirror.co.uk/news/top-stories/2009/08/09/swine-flu-kills-41st-uk-victim-115875-21583342/.
- "H1N1: Six more deaths recorded". News Straits Times. 2009-08-11. Retrieved on 2009-08-11.
- http://www.prensa-latina.cu/index.php?option=com_content&task=view&id=105945&Itemid=1.
- http://www.cre.com.ec/Desktop.aspx?Id=143&e=130919.
- "Pandemic Influenza (h1n1) 09 Swine Flu - Update 131". New Zealand MoH. 2009-08-11. Retrieved on 2009-08-11.
- "Sign of community spread". *Calcutta Telegraph*. 2009-08-11. Retrieved on 2009-08-11.

- "Sixth swine flu death in Pune, toll mounts to 12". *Times of India*. 2009-08-12. Retrieved on 2009-08-12.
- http://www.sns.gov.bo/snis/default.aspx.
- http://www.mspas.gob.sv/virus_gripeA_H1N1/boletines.htm.
- "Swine flu fatality rate rose to 6 in total". *GMANEWSTV*. 31 July 2009. Retrieved on 2009-07-31.
- Cimatu, Frank; Vincent Cabreza (29 July 2009). "Swine flu kills 4 in Cordilleras, 1 in HK". Inquirer Northern Luzon. Retrieved on 2009-07-29.
- "EISN Weekly electronic bulletin Week 31: 27 July 2009 - 02 August 2009". ECDC. 2009-08-07. Retrieved on 2009-08-07.
- "Spain announces 6th death of A/H1N1 flu". Xinhua. 2009-07-28. Retrieved on 2009-07-28.
- "Spain Records 9th Death From Swine Flu". *Wall Street Journal*. 2009-08-10. Retrieved on 2009-08-10.
- "Situational Update of Cases". Ministry of Health, Singapore. 2009-07-07. Retrieved on 2009-07-08.
- "Singapore reports one more A/H1N1 related death". Xinhua. 2009-08-09. Retrieved on 2009-08-09.
- "Latest situation in the Region". WHO. 2009-08-03. Retrieved on 2009-08-03.
- "H1N1 death toll up to 9". Saudi Gazette. 2009-08-10. Retrieved on 2009-08-10.
- "Honduras' confirmed A/H1N1 flu cases climb to 263". Xinhua. 2009-08-11. Retrieved on 2009-08-11.
- "Week 30: 20/07/2009-26/07/2009". *EuroFlu - Weekly Electronic Bulletin*. EuroFlu. 2009-07-31. Retrieved on 2009-07-31.
- http://www.almomento.net/news/127/ARTICLE/39822/2009-08-11.html.
- "Update on Human Swine Influenza" (PDF). Surveillance and Epidemiology Branch, Centre for Health Protection. 2009-08-10. Retrieved on 2009-08-10.
- "South Africans Panic As Swine Flu Cases Continue To Rise". Radio VOP. 2009-08-11. Retrieved on 2009-08-11.
- "Third swine flu death in SA". iol.co.za. 2009-08-11. Retrieved on 2009-08-11.
- "Toddler dies of suspected H1N1 as cases rise to 771". Jakarta Post. 2009-08-11. Retrieved on 2009-08-11.

- "Vietnam's A/H1N1 flu cases rise to over 1,200". Xinhua. 2009-08-11. Retrieved on 2009-08-11.
- http://www.xaluan.com/modules.php?name=News&file=article&sid=135213.
- Includes Aruba and the Netherlands Antilles.
- "Netherlands reports first death from H1N1 flu". Reuters. 2009-08-04. Retrieved on 2009-08-04.
- "Week 29 : 13/07/2009-19/07/2009". *EuroFlu - Weekly Electronic Bulletin*. EuroFlu. 2009-07-24. Retrieved on 2009-07-28.
- "Grippe A/H1N1 : Bulletin épidémiologique" (in French). French governement : Grippe A/H1N1 : Bulletin gripe du 22 juillet. 2009-07-22. Retrieved on 2009-07-26.
- "Egypt's A/H1N1 Flu Cases Reach 402". CRIEnglish. 2009-08-11. Retrieved on 2009-08-11.
- "Swine flu fears allayed, rumour-mongers warned". *Gulf Times*. 2009-08-11. Retrieved on 2009-08-11.
- "Regional Update Pandemic (H1N1) 2009. Qualitative Indicators by Epidemiological Week. Week 29." PAHO. Retrieved on 2009-08-03.
- "Situationseinschätzung zur Neuen Influenza" (in German). Robert Koch Institut. 2009-08-11. Retrieved on 2009-08-11.
- "Cases of Influenza A (H1N1) Virus in Japan". Ministry of Health, Labour and Welfare. 2009-07-24. Retrieved on 2009-07-24.
- "S. Korea confirms 51 more cases of influenza A". Yonhap. 2009-08-09. Retrieved on 2009-08-09.
- Localized spread in South Greece, according to WHO update 60.
- "Number of swine flu cases surpasses 1,000". Kathimerni. 2009-08-06. Retrieved on 2009-08-06.
- "Dynamisk Rapport" (in Norwegian). Peoples Health Institute (department MSIS Reporting System for Infectious Diseases). Retrieved on 2009-08-11.
- "H1N1 in Saudi Arabia". HC2D.co.uk. 2009-08-11. Retrieved on 2009-08-11.
- "Macao's A/H1N1 confirmed cases reach 300". *People's Daily Online*. 2009-08-11. Retrieved on 2009-08-11.
- "Panel plans new measures to tackle H1N1 spread". Zawya. 2009-08-11. Retrieved on 2009-08-11.
- "10/08/2009 Tarihli Açýklama".

- "EUROPEAN INFLUENZA SURVEILLANCE NETWORK". *Weekly electronic bulletin Week 29: 13 July 2009 - 19 July 2009*. ECDC. 2009-07-24. Retrieved on 2009-07-26.
- "Qatar swine flu victim 'fell ill in Dubai'". *The Naitonal*. 2009-08-01. Retrieved on 2009-08-01.
- "121 H1N1 cases reported in Serbia, Kosmet". emportal.rs. 2009-08-04. Retrieved on 2009-08-04.
- "Swine flu total reaches 99 as ministry launches awareness campaign". *Jordan Times*. 2009-08-05. Retrieved on 2009-08-05.
- "Morocco: seven new cases of swine influenza detected". Ennahar Online. 2009-08-11. Retrieved on 2009-08-11.
- Jersey and Guernsey are reported together by ECDC as 'Channel Islands'.
- "Macedonia confirms another two A type flu cases". MRT.com. 2009-08-05. Retrieved on 2009-08-05.
- "Algeria: a new case of swine flu identified". *Ennahar Online*. 2009-08-11. Retrieved on 2009-08-11.
- "Three more swine flu cases". MyRepublica.com. 2009-08-10. Retrieved on 2009-08-10.
- "Two more cases of disease of the influenza A (H1N1) confirmed in Kazakhstan". Gazeta.kz. 2009-08-06. Retrieved on 2009-08-06.
- "Influenza cases rise to 16 in Myanmar". *Trend.az*. 2009-08-09. Retrieved on 2009-08-09.
- "Yemen Records 13th Swine Flu Infection". *Yemen Post*. 2009-08-08. Retrieved on 2009-08-08.
- "Swine flu under control in Kosovo". EMPortal.rs. 2009-08-07. Retrieved on 2009-08-07.
- "Namibia: Swine Flu Spreads in Country". allafrica.com. 2009-08-10. Retrieved on 2009-08-10.
- "Two more test swine flu positive". *KuenseOnline*. 2009-08-07. Retrieved on 2009-08-07.
- "NMI swine flu cases now at 6". *Saipan Tribune*. 2009-08-04. Retrieved on 2009-08-04.
- "Zambia confirms five cases of A/H1N1 flu". Xinhua. 2009-07-29. Retrieved on 2009-07-29.
- "Regional Update Pandemic (H1N1) 2009". Paho. 209-07-22. Retrieved on 2009-07-25.
- http://www.chronicle.gi/headlines_details.php?id=16866.

- "Maldivian woman quarantined after testing positive for Influenza-A virus". haveeruonline.com.mv. 2009-08-10. Retrieved on 2009-08-10.
- "Situation updates - Influenza A(H1N1)". *Epidemic and Pandemic Alert and Response.* WHO. Retrieved on 2009-05-13.
- "Human infection with pandemic (H1N1) 2009 virus: updated interim WHO guidance on global surveillance". *Annex 4.* WHO. 2009-07-10. pp. 16. Retrieved on 2009-07-25.
- Dawood FS, Jain S, Finelli L, *et al.* (June 2009). "Emergence of a novel swine-origin influenza A (H1N1) virus in humans". *N. Engl. J. Med.* (25): 2605–15.doi:10.1056/NEJMoa0903810. PMID 19423869. "the number of confirmed cases is an underestimate of the number of cases that have occurred".
- CDC (12th March 2009). "Questions and Answers Regarding Estimating Deaths from Influenza in the United States". CDC.
- "Swine Flu Might Have Come From Asia" *New York Times,* June 23, 2009.
- "Pandemic (H1N1) 2009 briefing note 3" (in 2009-07-16). WHO. Retrieved on 2009-07-17.
- "W.H.O. Says It Plans to Stop Tracking Swine Flu Cases" *New York Times,* July 16, 2009.
- "CDC Briefing on Investigation of Human Cases of H1N1 Flu". CDC. 2009-07-24. Retrieved on 2009-07-28.
- *Flu Activity & Surveillance,* CDC.
- Jordan Ellenberg (4th July 2009). "Influenza Body Count". Slate.
- "Human infection with pandemic (H1N1) 2009 virus: updated interim WHO guidance on global surveillance". WHO. 2009-07-10. Retrieved on 2009-07-17.
- "New Push in H1N1 Flu Fight Set for Start of School" *Wall Street Journal,* July 18, 2009.
- Kurtz, Howard (27 April 2009). "Media's coverage of swine flu is feverish". Newsday. (from *The Washington Post*).
- Altman Lawrence K (28 April 2009). "Sound the alarm? A swine flu bind". New York Times. Retrieved on 2009-04-30.
- "GLOBAL: No A (H1N1) cases - reality or poor lab facilities?". Reuters. 8 May 2009. Retrieved on 9 May 2009.
- "When is a pandemic not a pandemic?" *Nature News,* May 21, 2009.
- "DRepublic denies it is under-reporting swine flu cases". ABS-CBN News. 31 May 2009.

- E. Eduardo Castillo (12 May 2009). "As swine flu spreads, who should get Tamiflu?". Associated Press.
- "School with swine flu case won't be named". Poughkeepsie, New York: Poughkeepsie Journal. 31 May 2009.
- "Swine Flu cases may have gone undetected" *Pro 8 News*, June 8, 2009.
- "Swine flu test results are unreliable, WHO warns" *The Sydney Morning Herald*, June 10, 2009.
- "Recent Utah Swine Flu Death May Have Been Preventable". 2009-06-24. Retrieved on 2009-07-16.
- "Influenza : Fact sheet". World Health Organization. March 2003. Retrieved on 2009-05-07.
- Kilbourne ED (January 2006). "Influenza pandemics of the 20th century.". *Emerging Infectious Diseases* (1).
- Hsieh, Yu-Chia; *et al.* (January 2006). "Influenza pandemics: past present and future" (PDF). *Journal of the Formosan Medical Association* (1): 1–6.
- "Finding the real case-fatality rate of H5N1 avian influenza". *J Epidemiol Community Health* (6): 555-559. 2008. doi:10.1136/jech.2007.064030. PMID 18477756.
- Knobler S, Mack A, Mahmoud A, Lemon S, ed. "1: The Story of Influenza". *The Threat of Pandemic Influenza: Are We Ready? Workshop Summary (2005).* Washington, D.C.: The National Academies Press. pp. 60–61.
- Patterson, KD; Pyle GF (Spring 1991). "The geography and mortality of the 1918 influenza pandemic". *Bull Hist Med.* (1): 4–21. PMID 2021692.
- "Ten things you need to know about pandemic influenza". World Health Organization. 14 October 2005.
- Taubenberger JK; Morens DM (January 2006). "1918 influenza: the mother of all pandemics". *Emerging Infectious Diseases* (Centers for Disease Control and Prevention).
- "WHO Europe - Influenza". World Health Organization. June 2009. Retrieved on 2009-06-12.
- David Brown (29 April 2009). "System set up after SARS epidemic was slow to alert global authorities". Washington Post.
- The Writing Committee of the World Health Organization (WHO) Consultation on Human Influenza A/H5 (September 2005). "Avian

influenza A (H5N1) infection in humans". *N Engl J Med*: 1374–85. doi:10.1056/NEJMra052211. PMID 16192482.

- McNeil Donald G Jr (May 20, 2009). "U.S. says older people appear safer from new flu strain". New York Times.
- Hayden Erica Check (5 May 2009). "The turbulent history of the A(H1N1) virus". *Nature*. Retrieved on 2009-05-07.
- Cohen Jon, Enserink Martin (1 May 2009). "As swine flu circles globe, scientists grapple with basic questions". Science.
- "Swine influenza A/Mexico/2009 (H1N1) update". 30 April 2009.
- "New flu has been around for years in pigs — study" *Reuters*, June 11, 2009.
- "Flu outbreak raises a set of questions". *New York Times*. April 26, 2009.
- "SWINE FLU: Mexico Faces Criticism Over Response" *Huffington Post*, April 27, 2009.
- "Swine flu: is intensive pig farming to blame?" *The Guardian*, April 28, 2009.
- "Flu crisis brought U.S., Mexico together" *Houston Chronicle*, June 6, 2009.
- "Study: Mexico has thousands more swine flu cases" *Chicago Sun-Times*, May 12, 2009.
- "Swine influenza A (H1N1) infection in two children — Southern California, March—April 2009". *Morbidity and Mortality Weekly Report*. Centers for Disease Control. April 22, 2009.
- Novel Swine-Origin Influenza A (H1N1) Virus Investigation Team (May 2009). "Emergence of a Novel Swine-Origin Influenza A (H1N1) Virus in Humans". *New England Journal of Medicine*. doi:10.1056/NEJMoa0903810. PMID 19423869.
- News report on confirmation of a new strain of flu in Mexico on 24 April 09 (in Spanish).
- "H1N1 virus genome: "This is a world first" *Independent*, May 6, 2009.
- "Fears of Avian Flu Said to Help U.S. Prepare for Swine Flu". *New York Times*. June 4, 2009.
- "Health officials evaluate response to swine flu" *Riverside Press-Enterprise*, June 7, 2009.
- "As swine flu wanes, U.S. preparing for second wave" *Reuters*, June 4, 2009.

- "Dealing with the Swine Flu Threat During Pregnancy" *U.S. News and World Report*, July 21, 2009.
- "Swine flu could kill hundreds of thousands in U.S. if vaccine fails, CDC says" *Los Angeles Times*, July 25, 2009.
- "Swine Flu: Why You Should Still Be Worried", *Fox News*, July 17, 2009.
- "Survey: Americans expect widespread swine flu" *Associated Press*, July 16, 2009.
- "Adverts promote swine flu service" *BBC*, July 24, 2009.
- "E.R.'s May Be the First Victims" *New York Times*, Aug. 2, 2009.
- "Swine flu goes to camp. Will it go to school next?" *Los Angeles Times*, July 27, 009.
- "The ABC's of H1N1" *New York Times*, Aug. 2, 2009.
- "Schools revamp swine flu plans for fall" *Houston Chronicle*, Aug. 1, 2009.
- "Fly the Germ-Free Skies" *New York Times*, Aug. 2, 2009.
- "Opnieuw twee gevallen van Mexicaanse griep in Belgie". Het Laatste Nieuws. 2009-05-15.
- "ECDC Situation Report 17 June 2009". European Centre for Disease Prevention and Control. 2009-06-17. Retrieved on 2009-06-17.
- "World now at the start of 2009 influenza pandemic". World Health Organization. 11 June 2009. Retrieved on 13 June 2009.
- "WHO - Influenza A(H1N1) - Travel". World Health Organization. 2009-05-07. Retrieved on 2009-06-17.
- "Swine flu travel warning lifted for Mexico", *Los Angeles Times*, May 15, 2009.
- *U.S. warns travelers about China's 7-day flu quarantine*, Seattle Times, June 22, 2009.
- Martin Andrew, Krauss Clifford (28 April 2009). "Pork industry fights concerns over swine flu". *The New York Times*.
- "EXCLUSIVE-WTO protectionism report to feature swine flu bans" *Reuters*, June 12, 2009.
- "US pork industry baffled by bans in China, Russia" *Associated Press*, May 4, 2009.
- "Pigs an underestimated source of flu: study" *Reuters*, June 4, 2009.
- CIDRAP news: Some immunity to novel H1N1 flu found in seniors, 21 May 2009.

- "Morbidity and Mortality Weekly Report Dispatch". U.S. Centers for Disease Control. 21 April 2009.
- Emma Wilkinson (2009-05-01). "What scientists know about swine flu". *BBC News*.
- Independent (May 6, 2009). "H1N1 virus genome: 'This is a world first'". Press release. Retrieved on May 6, 2009.
- Smith GJD, Vijaykrishna D, Bahl J, Lycett SJ, Worobey M, Pybus OG, Ma SK, Cheung CL, Raghwani J, Bhatt S, Peiris JSM, Guan Y & Rambaut A (11 June 2009). "Origins and evolutionary genomics of the 2009 swine-origin H1N1 influenza A epidemic". *Nature*. doi:10.1038/nature08182. Lay summary. (near-final letter).
- Davis, Mike. "The Swine Flu Crisis Lays Bare the Meat Industry's Monstrous Power" *Alternet.org*, April 28, 2009.
- "WHO: Swine Flu Could Infect 2 Billion" *CBS News*, July 24, 2009.
- "CDC Says Up to 24% of Americans Might Get Swine Flu if There Is No Vaccine" *WebMD*, July 24, 2009.
- "How many people have swine flu? No one knows" *Reuters*, July 24, 2009.
- "1 Million Americans Likely Stricken by Swine Flu: CDC" *Forbes*, June 25, 2009.
- "Swine flu is spreading more widely than official numbers show". *Bloomberg News*. 25May 2009.
- "UK swine flu toll is really 30,000, says leading scientist". *The Independent*. 24 May 2009.
- "Swine flu may have infected more than 100,000 Americans". *Atlanta Journal-Constitution*. 17 May 2009.
- "Swine flue may be scary, but 250 times as many die from regular flu" *New York Daily News*, June 7, 2009.
- "Figuring How to Terrify Us Over Swine Flu" *Townhall*, July 30, 2009.
- "WHO chief warns H1N1 swine flu likely to worsen". *Intellasia*. May 23, 2009.
- "New virus "very unstable", more changes seen-expert". *Reuters*. May 12, 2009.
- "Avian Influenza Disease Emergency Situation Update" (PDF). FAO. July 25, 2008.
- Steve Sternberg (May 26, 2009). "CDC expert says flu outbreak is dying down – for now".

- "CDC says no sign yet that swine flu is mutating" *Associated Press*, July 23, 2009.
- "WHO Pandemic Influenza Phases". World Health Organization. Retrieved on 2009-04-27.
- "Highlights of comments on flu by WHO chief Chan". *Reuters*. 11 June 2009.
- "Poor countries frontline of WHO pandemic flu battle" *Reuters*, June 12, 2009.
- CDC article *2008-2009 Influenza Season Week 21 ending May 30, 2009* Also see seasonal flu cases versus non-seasonal flu cases.
- WHO article *Transcript of virtual press conference with* Dr Keiji Fukuda, Assistant Director-General ad Interim for Health Security and Environment, World Health Organization *7 July 2009*.
- "CDC says swine flu has peaked in Mexico" *Associated Press*, June 4, 2009.
- World Health Organization Official: Swine Flu Close to Becoming Global Pandemic, Latina, Akanke Small, June 4, 2009.
- WHO official says world edging towards pandemic, Reuters, Laura MacInnis and Stephanie Nebehay, June 2, 2009.
- "INFORME SITUACIÓN DE INFECCIÓN POR NUEVA INFLUENZA A (H1N1) EN CHILE AL 19 DE JUNIO DE 2009". 2009-06-19. Retrieved on 2009-06-19.
- "Melbourne 'world's swine flu capital' " *SBS TV*, June 6, 2009.
- "Tough tests skewing swine flu figures: expert" *ABC News*, June 8, 2009.
- "Swine flu detected at Argentina pig farm" *Associated Press*, June 26, 2009.
- "No eran 1.587, sino más de 100 mil los contagiados" *Crítica Digital*, July 3, 2009.
- "'First' swine-flu death in Africa'". BBC News. August 3, 2009. Retrieved on 2009-08-05.
- Centers for Disease Control and Prevention (CDC) article *Interim Guidance for H1N1 Flu (Swine Flu): Taking Care of a Sick Person in Your Home* updated regularly.
- "What to do if you get flu-like symptoms". Centers for Disease Control and Prevention. 2009-05-07. Retrieved on 2009-05-22.
- "About the disease". World Health Organization. 2009-05-01. Retrieved on 2009-05-22.
- Emergence of a Novel Swine-Origin Influenza A (H1N1) Virus in

Humans, New England Journal of Medicine, May 7, 2009. Republished June 18. The study ran from April 15 through May 5. Patients with confirmed swine flu, and among patients for whom clinical information was available, 371 out of 394 (94%) had fever, and 365 out of 397 (92%) had cough.

- " 'Underlying conditions' may add to flu worries". *New York Times*. 27 May 2009.
- "Flu Pandemic Spurs Queries About Vaccine" *Wall Street Journal*, June 15, 2009.
- "New York City officials struggle for balanced response to swine flu". *Los Angeles Times*. 21 May 2009.
- "Spread of Swine Flu Puts Japan in Crisis Mode". *New York Times*. 21 May 2009.
- "Japanese schools reopen as swine flu threat abates". *Bloomberg News*. 23 May 2009.
- "Mexico City ends swine flu alert, no cases in week". *Associated Press*. 21 May 2009.
- "A new symptom of swine flu: seizures" *Los Angeles Times*, July 24, 2009.
- "Swine flu cases climbing". Foodconsumer.com. 30 May 2009.
- "Swine flu: U.S. sees new deaths in multiple states as Mexico may have passed peak" *Chicago Tribune*, June 5, 2009.
- Parker A. Small, Jr., M.D. and Bradley S. Bender, M.D. "Influenza: A to B". University of Florida Continuing Medical Education.
- Donald G. McNeil, Jr. (2009-05-18). "Other Illness May Precede Worst Cases of Swine Flu".
- "Viral Infections Followed by Bacterial Pneumonia". University of Florida Continuing Medical Education.
- "Most Deaths In 1918 Influenza Pandemic Caused By Bacterial Pneumonia". *Medical News Today*. 2008-08-20.
- "Vaccine for bacterial pneumonia does double duty". 2004-07-12.
- "Flu Prevention" Mayo Clinic.
- "Face masks aren't a sure bet against swine flu". *Los Angeles Times*. 30 April 2009.
- http://news.bbc.co.uk/2/hi/uk_news/8024690.stm.
- CDCRetrieved June 11, 2009.
- "A New Pandemic Fear: A Shortage of Surgical Masks" *Time*, May 19, 2009.

- CDC (2009-07-21). "CDC Director's Update Brief". (Republication of an unofficial document; confirmed at).
- "Joint FAO/WHO/OIE Statement on influenza A (H1N1) and the safety of pork". Press release. 7 May 2009.
- "No more pillows, blankets on Alaska Airlines" *Puget Sound Business Journal*, May 4, 2009.
- "Global airlines move to reduce infection risks" *Reuters*, June 3, 2009.
- "'Too late' to contain swine flu". *BBC News*. 28 April 2009. Retrieved on 28 April 2009.
- "Travel warning: Novel H1N1 flu and severe cases of respiratory illness in Mexico —Avoid nonessential travel to Mexico". Centers for Disease Control and Prevention. 30 April 2009. Retrieved on 6 May 2009.
- "Press Briefing Transcript —ogr. Media availability on CDC investigation of human cases of swine influenza". Centers for Disease Control and Prevention. 25 April 2009. Retrieved on 26 April 2009.
- "Expert: New strain of swine flu here to stay". *West Palm Beach News* (WPTV). 29 April 2009. Retrieved on 2 May 2009.
- "China quarantines U.S. school group over flu concerns". *CNN*. 28 May 2009.
- *Travel Advisories*, State Department.
- "Nagin's Phone Calls Screened 'to Keep Him Safe' While Quarantined in China" *Fox News*, June 8, 2009.
- "Caught in China's aggressive swine flu net". 29 May 2009.
- "Ship passengers cruisy in swine flu quarantine". Australian Broadcasting Corporation. 28 May 2009.
- "Egypt warns of post-hajj swine flu quarantine". Associated Press. 20 May 2009.
- "Swine flu prompts EU warning on travel to U.S.". Associated Press. 27 April 2009.
- "Marine with swine flu prompts quarantine". MSNBC. 29 April 2009.
- "Japan: swine flu quarantine ends for Air Passengers". NTDTV Japan TV. 15 May 2009.
- "Mongolia quarantines air passengers following swine flu alert" *Mongolia-Web*, May 7, 2009.

- "11 swine flu cases in India; don't panic, says government" *The Medguru*, June 8, 2009.
- "Egypt quarantines university dorm over swine flu" *Al Arabiya News Channel*, June 8, 2009.
- "New Orleans Mayor Quarantined By Chinese" *RTT News*, June 8, 2009.
- "Swine flu scare at university dorm in Cairo" *BBC News*, June 8, 2009.
- "Govt boosts powers to control swine flu" *New Zealand Herald*, June 8, 2009.
- Swine flu cases in India cross 500-mark.
- "India wants US to screen passengers for swine flu" *Sindh Today*, June 16, 2009.
- *Bay Area records first death tied to swine flu*, June 6, 2009.
- *NY schools back on track after swine flu*, *Newsday*, June 5, 2009.
- "Swine Flu's Presence Poses Tough Choices For School Officials" *Hartford Courant*, June 6, 2009.
- "Teachers' union worried about swine flu school closures" *ABC News*, June 4, 2009.
- "Philippines postpones classes because of swine flu" *Philstar.com*, June 6, 2009.
- "WHO Declares Swine Flu Pandemic" *Time CNN*, June 11, 2009.
- South China Morning Post, "Schools on standby for flu closure", 11 June, 2009.
- "Schools closed in Guatemala.", 10 June, 2009.
- "Buenos Aires brings forward school vacations". *Buenos Aires Herald*, 30 June, 2009.
- *Dan una semana más de vacaciones en Costa Rica por influenza humana* (in Spanish), SDP Noticias, 2009-07-13.
- Dan una semana más de vacaciones en Costa Rica por influenza humana.
- http://www.hse.gov.uk/news/2009/swineflu.htm Retrieved on 5 July 2009.
- "WHO: No licensed swine flu vaccine til end of year" *Associated Press*, July 13, 2009.
- "Preparing for the worst". *The Economist*. 7 May 2009.
- "Fight for swine flu vaccine could get ugly" *Associated Press*, July 16, 2009.

- *Swine Flu Vaccinations to be Expedited in Europe*, RedOrbit.com, July 26, 2009.
- "H1N1 vaccine may not be ready in time for fall" *Baltimore Sun*, June 15, 2009.
- "First defense against swine flu—seasonal vaccine" *Reuters*, July 24, 2009.
- "Swine Flu Multiple-Shot Vaccine May Overwhelm States" *Bloomberg News*, June 26, 2009.
- Mayo Clinic Staff. "Influenza (flu) treatments and drugs". *Diseases and Conditions*. Mayo Clinic. Retrieved on 20 May 2009.
- Macdonald S (2002). "Aspirin use to be banned in under 16 year olds". *BMJ* 325 (7371): 988. doi:10.1136/bmj.325.7371.988/c. PMID 12411346.
- "Fever". *Medline Plus Medical Encyclopedia*. U.S. National Library of Medicine. Retrieved on 20 May 2009.
- "What to do if you get flu-like symptoms". Centers for Disease Control and Prevention. 7 May 2009. Retrieved on 20 May 2009.
- "Tamiflu-Resistant Swine Flu in U.S.?", *WebMD*, July 7, 2009.
- Declan Butler (14 May 2009). "Marie-Paule Kieny : The vaccine research director of the World Health Organization, on swine flu". Nature News. doi:10.1038/news.2009.478.
- "How a Mild Virus Might Turn Vicious". *New York Times*. June 8, 2009.
- "Warning against buying flu drugs online". *The Guardian*. 8 May 2009.
- "Swine Flu: A Wake-up Call for Emergency Planners" *IT World*, June 8, 2009.
- "Criminals may exploit swine flu pandemic" *WA Today - Australia*, June 10, 2009.
- "Bandits Steal 75,000 Salk Shots As Montreal Fights Polio Wave", *New York Times*, Sept. 1, 1959.
- "FDA campaign against swine flu scams making a dent" *Associated Press*, June 15, 2009.
- "US looks to change 'swine flu' name". Agence France-Presse. 29 April 2009. Retrieved on 2009-04-29.
- "H1N1 Flu". Centers for Disease Control and Prevention.
- "South Korea changed the name 'swine flu' to 'Mexican virus'". BCC (Taiwan). 29 April 2009. (Traditional Chinese).

- "Renamed swine flu certain to hit Taiwan". *The China Post*. 29 April 2009.
- Bradsher Keith (28 April 2009). "The naming of swine flu, a curious matter". *New York Times*. Retrieved on 2009-04-29.
- Pilkington Ed (28 April 2009). "What's in a name? Governments debate 'swine flu' versus 'Mexican' flu". *The Guardian*. Retrieved on 29 April 2009.
- "Stick to Name 'Swine Flu,' WHO Says as Industry Moans". *Bloomberg*. 28 April 2009.
- "Epidemic and pandemic alert and response (EPR)". *World Health Organization*. Retrieved on 1 May 2009.
- World Health Organization (30 April 2009). "Joint FAO/WHO/OIE statement on influenza A(H1N1) and the safety of pork". Press release. Retrieved on 1 May 2009.
- "WHO changes swine flu name to 'H1N1 influenza', 257 confirmed cases". DPA. *Hindustan Times*. 30 April 2009. Retrieved on 2 May 2009.
- "[Not swine nor Mexican, the WHO baptises the flu with 'H1']" (in Spanish). Madrid: ABC Periódico Electrónico. 1 May 2009. Retrieved on 2 May 2009.
- "Name dilemma: Swine flu or Mexican flu?" *India Times*. 30 April 2009.
- "Update: infections with a swine-origin influenza A (H1N1) virus - United States and other countries". *Morbidity and Mortality Weekly Report* (U.S. Centers for Disease Control). 28 April 2009.

Index